First Aid
and
Emergency
Nursing

First Aid
and
Emergency
Nursing

NN Yalayyaswamy MSc (N), DN (Ed)
Former Professor of Nursing
Government College of Nursing
Bangalore

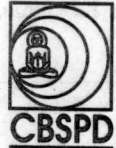

CBS Publishers & Distributors Pvt Ltd

New Delhi • Bengaluru • Chennai • Kochi • Kolkata • Lucknow • Mumbai
Gujarat • Hyderabad • Jharkhand • Nagpur • Patna • Pune • Uttarakhand

First Aid
and
Emergency
Nursing

ISBN: 978-81-239-1668-2

CBS Reprint: 2009, 2010, 2011, 2012, 2014, 2016, 2018, 2021, 2022, 2024, **2026**
First Edition: 1997
Reprint: 1998, 1999, 2002, 2004

Published by **Satish Kumar Jain** and produced by **Varun Jain** for

CBS Publishers & Distributors Pvt Ltd

4819/XI Prahlad Street, 24 Ansari Road, Daryaganj, New Delhi 110 002, India.
Ph: 011-23266838, 23289259   Website: www.cbspd.corn
e-mail: delhi@cbspd.com

Corporate Office: 204 FIE, Industrial Area, Patparganj, Delhi 110 092
Ph: 011-4934 4934   Fax: 011-4934 4935
e-mail: publishing@cbspd.com; publicity@cbspd.com

Branches

- **Bengaluru:** Seema House 2975, 17th Cross, KR Road, Banasankari 2nd Stage, Bengaluru 560 070,
  Karnataka, India
  Ph: +91-80-26771678/79   Fax: +91-80-26771680   e-mail: bangalore@cbspd.com
- **Chennai:** 18/8B, Subbaraya Street, Shenoy Nagar, Chennai 600 030, Tamil Nadu, India
  Ph: +91-044-42032115, 044-26681266   e-mail: chennai@cbspd.com
- **Kochi:** 42/1325, 1326, Power House Road, Opp KSEB, Power House, Ernakulum Kochi 682 018,
  Kerala, India
  Ph: +91-484-4059061-65,67   Fax: +91-484-4059065   e-mail: kochi@cbspd.com
- **Kolkata:** 147, Hind Ceramics Compound, 1st Floor, Nilgunj Road, Belghoria, Kolkata-700056, West
  Bengal, India
  Ph: +033-25633055, 033-25633056   e-mail: kolkata@cbspd.com
- **Lucknow:** Basement, Khushnuma Complex, 7 Meerabai Marg (Behind Jawahar Bhawan),
  Lucknow-226001, UP, India
  Ph: +0522-4000032   e-mail: tiwari.lucknow@cbspd.com
- **Mumbai:** PWD Shed, Gala no 25/26, Ramchandra Bhatt Marg, Next to JJ Hospital Gate no. 2, Opp.
  Union Bank of India, Noorbaug, Mumbai-400009, Maharashtra, India
  Ph: 022-66661880/89   e-mail: mumbai@cbspd.com

Representatives

- Gujarat · 0-9879558667
- Nagpur   0-8692091830
- Uttarakhand 0-9716462459
- Hyderabad 0-9885175004
- Patna 0-9334159340
- Jharkhand 0-9811541605
- Pune 0-9664372571

Printed at Glorious Printers, Jhilmil Industrial Area, Delhi, India

PREFACE

The new text book on **"First Aid and Emergency Nursing"** have been exclusively developed for the use of nursing and other paramedical professionals. This book is also designed, keeping in view the current syllabus of General Nursing and Midwifery Course.

First Aid is a subject to be known by a common man to meet the urgent needs of a victim in case of accidents and other natural calamities. In the present society as the life-style changes to suit the new environment, one is bound to come across various episodes which require an urgent attention. If a person who attends to such type of victims, probably will be in a position to save the life. The commonest conditions such as broken bones and heart attacks usually leads to complications, which if neglected may end in disastrous state. Hence, if a first-aider comes to first help, probably the life could be saved or atleast will be able to guide the victim to the nearest medical help.

I hope this book will meet the requirements of first-aider, practicing within the profession as well as a literate general public.

I thank M/s. Gajanana Book Publishers & Distributors for undertaking this publication and M/s. Typograph for their excellent typesetting and graphic work.

Bangalore   N. N. Yalayyaswamy

January 14, 1997

CONTENTS

FIRST AID AND EMERGENCY NURSING

Introduction

What is First aid?

If any person suffers an accident or any sudden disease, the aid that can be given by those who are near him before taking him to a doctor, is called First Aid. First aid is a most important branch of medical science, one in which a lay man has a useful and rewarding part to play. It requires progressive acquirement of learning and skill. An organised worldwide effort came in 187, though First aid was being practiced from ancient times. It was the famous German Surgeon who first conceived the idea of "First aid". He was General Esmarch (1823-1908). In 1877 St. John Ambulance Association of England was formed. In 1920, Red Cross Society of India was established. With more than 400 branches all over India, great success has been achieved in the improvement of health and prevention of diseases.

This is an age when technology has produced complicated machinery and swift means of transport. So, accidents are on the rise and produce devastating results with loss of life, injuries to body and mind. Under these circumstances, first aid has gained much importance. First aid can also be defined as the immediate and temporary care given to an injured or sick person until the services of a qualified Doctor are obtained. Proper and immediate care is absolutely necessary to save life and mitigate suffering. The First aid is not an end by itself. It indicates that the person is in need of a "Secondary Aid".

What are the objects of First Aid?

First aid is, mainly, based on the knowledge of human anatomy and physiology. It can be a life saving skill. The main objects of first aid are:

1. **To save life :** It should ensure that the adverse effects of injury are controlled, breathing and heart beat are restored to normal levels and bleeding, if any, controlled. As a whole, the immediate objects of first aid at a given situation is to save the life of the individual.

2. **To ease the pain :** When a patient is suffering from great pain due to the accident, it is the first object of first aid to reduce pain and prevent further injury or complication. It should be ensured that does not worsen. It should promote recovery of injured parts speedily.

3. **To avoid further injury :** First aid should help to avoid further injury. It should correct situations which tend to increase the original injury.

4. **Prepare for medical treatment :** This is done first by arranging suitable mode of transport to take the patient to the hospital. The First aid should form a basis for subsequent treatment by the doctor or the hospital staff.

2

5. **To assist the Doctor** : It can be done by supplying details of accident, injury and the first aid treatment given etc.,

The ultimate aim of First aid is to prevent disability and death.

To obtain understanding of the working of the human body and its response to injury and illness. This would be a good introduction to the study of medical science in a practical way.

What are the limitations of First aid (Scope)?

The first aider should reach the place of the accident quickly. He should be cool and calm and get on with his work, methodically. First, he should inspire confidence in the patient and others closely related to the patient. If the casualty is handled clumsily, it may cause greater harm and even cause death. Any attempt at more ambitious treatment may easily prove more harmful than the original injury.

To save lives, there are three conditions that call for first aid. They are stoppage of breathing, severe bleeding and shock. If breathing movements are not proper, the lips, tongue and finger nails become blue. In such a situation, artificial respiration should be started immediately. If there is heavy bleeding, it may be from wounds through one or more large vessels. Such a loss of blood can cause death with in a few minutes. So, we should not waste time. Pressure should be applied directly over the wound. A clean hand kerchief or a pad may be kept on the wound and pressed firmly with one or both hands, then apply a firm bandage. Keep the bleeding part higher than the rest of the body.

The third important factor to be attended immediately is shock. This is called "illness of injury" and requires treatment of the patient as a whole and not

3

the injury itself. Shock accompanies severe injury or emotional disturbance. Cold and clammy skin, beads of perspiration on the forehead and palms. Pale face, nausea and vomiting are the common symptoms of shock.

It is not the responsibility of the First aider to conclude that death has taken place. Some times, it is difficult even for a doctor to define the time of death. So, the first aider should not assume death until the doctor arrives and declares that the patient is dead.

First take the casualty away from fire, live wires, moving machinery etc. Keep the patient in a safe and clear place. Do not allow people to crowd around the casualty. If the weather is extremely· cold or hot or it is raining heavily, take the patient to a near by room or a sheltered place. If there is no such facility, make use of an umbrella or a newspaper etc. The injured person should be made lying in a comfortable position on his back. His belt should be loosened, open the buttons of his shirt and trousers. Keep his legs in a natural position with toes facing up. The injured person should be kept comfortable but not hot. Water or other liquids should not be given to an unconscious person. The person should not be allowed to see his own injury. If there are wounds on the body, they should be cleaned gently and then dressed. In the case of burn victims, their clothes should not be pulled out. They should be cut with a clean scissors and removed. If there is bleeding, stop bleeding by pressure bandage.

Use soft words and reassure the casualty. Send the patient to a hospital or a doctor by quickest means of transport. Inform the relatives of the patient, if possible. Always remember that you are only a first aider and not a doctor. Only as much assistance as is necessary to save life, should be given.

What are the principles of emergency care?

1. Obtain a correct and detailed history of accident either from the patient or any one who saw the accident.

2. The injured person may be examined thoroughly, taking note of every symptom. Only then you can make a diagnosis.

3. With the help of the above diagnosis, treat the casualty until the doctor arrives or the patient is shifted to a hospital. First aid is necessary during this intervening period.

4. It is always better to shift the patient to a hospital or call a doctor as soon as possible. Treatment from a doctor provides a better chance of recovery than prolonging the first aid.

If the accident occurs at home and there is nobody at home, call the neighbour for help. If the accident occurs in a public place, call the police. It is always better to keep the phone numbers of your doctor, police control room, fire brigade, local hospital with you. Any of them may be contacted during an emergency. As soon as possible, a message can be sent to the relatives as to the condition of the patient and the address of the hospital or doctor, he is being taken to. If first aid kits are available, use them efficiently.

What are considered as golden rules of First aid?

1. Be calm and quick. Be methodical. Patiently, find out all major injuries and wounds and treat them suitably.

2. In case of stoppage of breathing, start artificial respiration.

3. Try to stop bleeding as early as possible.

4. Do not allow a patient to go with a shock. If it is not possible, transport the patient to a near by hospital as quickly as possible

5. Keep the patient warm and do not move him unnecessarily. Keep him in a comfortable position.

6. Do only what is necessary.

7. Reassure the casualty by using encouraging words and obtain the help of his relatives.

8. Do not allow people to crowd around the casualty. Allow fresh air.

9. Be careful in removing his clothes. Do not cause injury. Keep the body warm and avoid shock. Send the patient to a doctor or a hospital by the quickest means of transport. When serious accident takes place, inform the police.

Points to remember

1. First aid is the immediate and effective service rendered to an injured sick person before the arrival of a doctor or shifted to a nearby hospital.

2. The main objects of First aid are to save life, to reduce or relieve pain, to avoid further injury, to set right the situations that might increase the original injury or illness and prevent disability and death.

3. To give efficient first aid, one should have good knowledge of anatomy and physiology of the human body and common sense and experience.

4. The first aider should be observant, tactful, resourceful, explicit and discriminating.

CASUALTY MANAGEMENT

When a first aider is called to attend an accident victim, he must consider many important details and also select the method to adopt which would decide the future welfare of society.

1. When an accident occurs at home or at school, there will be several facilities for treatment. There is no hurry and first aid can be planned methodically.

   But, if the accident occurs in a street, the method should be suitably altered according to the facilities available. Delay is harmful and the patient should be transported to the nearest hospital. So, our approach and method of first aid depends on the circumstances and the place of the accident.

2. When the first aider comes to know about the accident and his services are needed, he should reach the spot of the accident as quickly as possible. While doing so, he should keep in mind of his physical limitations. If he reaches the spot breathless and needs rest for a few minutes, it would delay the first aid and that may prove very costly. So, deliberate approach is necessary.

3. Before starting first aid, permission should be obtained either from the patient or his close relatives.

4. When once the permission is obtained, he should observe the patient from some distance and notice the circumstances under which the accident occurred. He should examine the need for any life saving measures, like artificial respiration etc.

5. When the first aider reaches the spot of the accident, the causes of the accident may still be present and continues to exert harmful effects. So, whenever possible, the cause of the accident must be removed without any delay. When it is not possible, the patient must be moved quickly. Then a quick examination of the patient should be made to detect the injuries.

6. The sources of danger which may cause further harm to the patient and also, the first aider should be considered and suitable steps taken to prevent this.

7. Sometimes, due to severe injury, the patient may appear collapsed and has lost the will to recover. This is called "Shock" and needs immediate treatment. The patient's confidence in his recovery must be ensured.

8. What treatment can be given and the amount of treatment, depends on the circumstances and facilities available at the spot of the accident. Every case must be considered on its own merits and separate treatment given according to the need.

9. If there are a number of casualties at a spot, the first aider must first examine each patient and decide on the order in which they are to be treated and shifted to a hospital. Treatment should start from the more severe patient to a lesser one. Stoppage of breathing, haemorrhage and general condition of the patient, require urgent care.

10. Seeking medical aid, depends on the circumstances and the decision should be taken at the earliest. When the accident has occurred in doors, the doctor should be sent for, as early as possible, so that, removal of the patient can be delayed until the patient has sufficient by recovered.

11. Bystanders can be made use of, to assist the first aider and also to send for bringing the doctor and to control on coming traffic and regulate the crowd Further assistance can be obtained through these by standers.

12. Removal of the patient to a hospital before any doctor's services can be procured, depends on the environment and the general conditions of the patient.

Handling and Transport

Loading a stretcher

Five people will be required to load a casualty on to a stretcher. Four to lift the casualty and one, to move the stretcher.

Fold the canvas sheet into a concertina shape. Make three complete folds from the top and four from the bottom. Slide the folded canvas under the casualty through the hollow of his back or adopt the procedure for a blanket lift.

Each person should place one foot on the top pile of folds, pull the casualty's clothing out from his waist down and gently work the canvas down under his buttocks and legs. Same thing is repeated for the top part of his body until the canvas is extended.

Starting from the casualty's head, slide the poles into the sleeves and place spacer bars over the ends if they are to be used.

Blanket lift

Two bearers should stand facing each other on either side of casualty's trunk and the two, face each other at his lower limbs. The two edges of the blanket may be rolled tightly up, against his side. The edges of the blanket can be rolled around them, if poles of sufficient length and rigidity are available. It would make the casualty easier to lift and prevent the blanket sagging.

With backs straight, squat and grasp the blanket with your palms downwards and fingers at the inner side of the rolled blanket edge.

The two bearers nearest to the casualty's head should each place one hand level with his head and the other at his waist. The bearers at the lower limbs should place one hand level with his hips and the other at his ankles. Working together lean back, and carefully and evenly lower the casualty on to the stretcher.

If a fifth person is not available or if it is not possible to push the stretcher under the casualty, place the stretcher in line with him as close to his head as possible. Carefully lift him and move with short even side paces until he is directly over the stretcher. Afterwards lower him on to it.

Manual lift for a fractured spine

If the casualty has a fractured spine, do not move him unless absolutely necessary. Sometimes you may have to lift the casualty on to a stretcher. When scoop stretcher cannot be used because of

1. soft ground

2. ambulance cannot reach the site of the accident

3. if danger dictates emergency movement, manual lift becomes necessary.

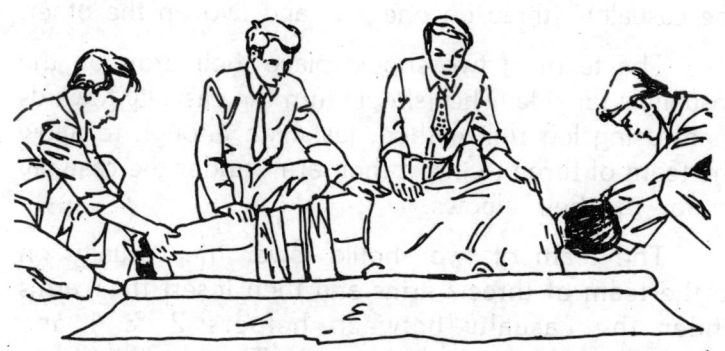

Figure 1. Position of helpers for manual lift

One person should kneel at the casualty's head and support his head and neck in the normal neutral position. Remove hard objects from his pockets. Put sufficient soft padding between his legs. Tie a figure of eight bandage around his knees. Place his arms across his chest.

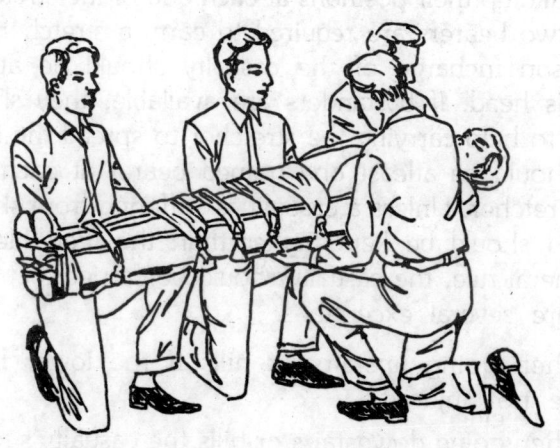

Figure 2. Manual lift for a fractured spine

11

Five helpers are necessary. They should remove all rings, watches etc. Then kneel on their right knees beside the casualty - three on one side and two on the other.

The team of two should place their arms on the casualty's far side. They should turn the casualty towards them using log roll method, just high enough to allow the team of three to insert their arms under the casualty as far as their elbows.

The team of two should lower the casualty on to the team of three's arms and then insert their arms under the casualty between helpers 2 & 4 and 4 & 6. Do not cross or hold hands. Then on the orders of the head holder, gently and evenly lift the casualty high enough to let the stretcher in.

A prepared stretcher should be placed under the casualty by other helpers. Working together, gently lower the casualty on to the stretcher, so that, his head is just clear of the top traverse. Remove your hands carefully.

Carrying a stretcher

After placing the casualty on the stretcher, the bearers should take up their positions at each end of the stretcher. Atleast two bearers are required to carry a stretcher and the person incharge of the casualty should be at the casualty's head. If bystanders are available, they should be used to help carrying the stretcher to spread the load. There should be atleast one trained bearer at each end of the stretcher. Unless a casualty is suffering from shock, the head should be kept higher than the feet. Hence, as a general rule, the casualty should be carried feet first. There are several exceptions.

1. When going upstairs or hills if the lower limbs are not injured.

2. When going downstairs or hills the casualty's lower limbs are injured or the casualty is suffering from hypothermia.

3. When carrying a casualty to the side or foot of a bed

4. When loading casualty into an ambulance.

Loading ambulance

Some ambulances have flat built in beds with grooves to take the runners of a standard stretcher. There should be 4 people to load this ambulance. One would stand inside the ambulance, ready to guide the stretcher. The other three would stand one on either side of the stretcher and one at the end, ready to lift. If there are two berths always load, the left one first.

If a trolley bed should be loaded into an ambulance, two bearers should take up their positions one at each side of the trolley bed. Raise the trolley bed to the required height by working together and feed or push it into the ambulance with head first.

Unloading an ambulance

One bearer takes hold of the handles at the back while another bearer holds the handles at the head in the ambulance. The bearer at the back, gently withdraws the stretcher or trolley bed. As this is done, two bearers, one on each side of the trolley bed, support it, moving with sides paces until the end is clear of the ambulance. Then the bearer gets down from the ambulance, takes the handles at the head and helps to lower the trolley bed or stretcher to the ground.

Points to remember

Casualty management can be organised according to environment, approach, arrival, permission, examination, removal of the cause sources of danger, scope of treatment, casualty care, multiple casualties medical aid, use of bystanders, removal, relationship with police and means of transport.

PROMOTING SAFETY CONSCIOUSNESS

1. Safety in the home

The cause of accidents is, generally, carelessness, quickness and tiredness. It is possible to avoid most of the accidents by taking quick and proper decisions. By following safety rules, most of the accidents can be avoided.

When there is any question of safety at home, the first thing to see, how strong and durable the house is and whether it is a safe place to live in. It is possible to control the bigger accidents by following safety measures:

1. Avoid stains of oil, grease etc. on cement, tiles or linoleum floor. Otherwise, there is every possibility of slipping and fracturing buttocks, legs or wrist.

2. Before going to bath, be sure that the floor of the bathroom is not slippery. Be careful, to see that you are not injured while taking a bath under a tap. If you are taking hot water bath, be sure, by putting your finger tip under water, that the water is not too hot.

3. During rainy season, if the windows do not open easily, do not try to open it by using your fist. The glass may break and cause injury to your fist. The frame should be pushed from upper side and down side. While using a gas stove in the kitchen, the switch should be put off properly after the work is over. When you are putting on the switch, the matchstick should be burnt immediately.

4. While using electrical appliances, always remember to separate the plug from their sockets. Otherwise, the plug of the mixer or grinder or iron box fixed in the socket is dangerous to children. Electrical appliances should not be touched with wet hands. Do not try to repair electrical appliances without removing the plug from the socket.

5. If you have a pistol, keep it always in the lock. Keep it empty.

6. Children should not have access to matchbox, medicines, germicides etc.

7. While taking out things from the higher level, do not use loosely fitted stools. Avoid sitting on a broken or loosely fitted chair.

8. Keep the toys of children in right place. Be sure that there is no possibility of these toys falling on your feet and injuring it.

9. Let the furniture of the house be in proper places. Otherwise, it may cause injury. Things used regularly should be kept in suitable places.

10. Do not search things in the dark. Torch or bed switch can be used. When you go out in the evening, keep the lights of the outer room on, so that, when you return, it would be easier to get in to the house.

15

11. When some pictures are to be hung on the wall, make sure the hooks and nails are properly fixed.

12. Lighted bulb should not be removed without the help of a cloth.

13. Do not stretch your ankles or stand on ankles when trying to take out something from the upper level.

14. While lifting anything from the floor do not bend down by the waist line. Bend the knees. If the object is heavy, do not lift by yourself, take the help of others.

15. When the doors of the house open to the innerside, open them slowly as there is the possibility of somebody standing behind the door.

16. The pot containing drinking water, should be covered properly.

Smoking

It is not only bad for health of the individual who smokes but also a dangerous fire hazard for others. The tip of a burning cigarette is as hot as 400°C. So, any combustible material coming in contact with it, catches fire immediately. We have seen many major fires being produced by this smoking. Inspite of knowing this danger, people smoke. Such fires can be avoided if these safe smoking practices are followed. Keep sufficient ash trays in the house. The ash tray may be filled with little water or sand to extinguish the cigarette. Paper or crash should not be put in the ash tray. Do not throw cigarettes into trash cans as they may contain oily rags and paper. If you are going out of the room even for a short while, do not leave a burning cigarette in the tray. if it falls, off it may cause major fire in the house. So, before putting a cigarette into the ash tray, extinguish it. Avoid smoking in bed or at any other place when you are sleepy. Within a few minutes after the cigarette falls on the pillow or mattress, the whole bedroom may go up in flames. Smoking in the kitchen when the gas stove is on is also equally dangerous.

It is best to avoid smoking but if it is not possible, atleast follow some of the precautions mentioned above.

Safety measures outside the home

Accidents occur not only inside the house but also outside the house, like school, playground and streets. Children at school should be careful to avoid these accidents. Teachers and parents should instruct the children regarding the safety measures to be taken while at school or play ground. The management of these institutions should also provide suitable building and furniture for the children. They should not be made to carry heavy bags as they cause injury to the neck and back of the children. The black board should be good and the teacher should write boldly on the black board, so that, there would be no strain on the eyes. The teacher should not, generally, use the cane but even when punishment is given, it should be given in such a way that child is not physically hurt. While making children to do physical exercise, the instructor should not give the same exercise to all the children, irrespective of their age and physical abilities. Instruction should be individual and not collective. Children should be advised to be careful while crossing roads and always walk on footpaths. If footpaths are not there, they should walk along right edge of the road.

From the time the child leaves the house till he or she returns home, all precautions should be meticulously taken to avoid accidents.

Roadside accidents are equally common and they can be avoided only by following the traffic rules. Vehicle drivers should follow their driving code. They should be alert about the mistakes of others and should be

17

alert to avoid accidents. Let them not think about who is wrong and who is right. They should know the traffic rules. They should have concern for the other road users, particularly, pedestrians. They should respect the right of others in using the road.

In general, some of these safety measures may be helpful in preventing accidents.

a) When you are walking, strolling and running be careful about the ditches, stones, peels of banana etc. which may cause slipping. During rainy season, walk carefully on the wet roads.

b) You must always look forward and below on the road to avoid accidents due to ditch or vehicles, coming from the opposite side. You must have a torch while walking in the dark.

c) Make use of the foot path while walking on the road. If there is no foot path, be careful about the traffic coming from the opposite side. Even, when you are right and the other one is wrong, be calm, and explain the traffic rules to the other person patiently. Do not quarrel.

d) When you are crossing the road, be careful about the traffic signals. When you are crossing the road, if you hear the siren of an ambulance or a police van, go back to the foot path immediately and keep on walking until these vehicles pass off.

e) When you are driving a vehicle, do not try to overtake any other vehicle. Wait for the side or signal from the opposite direction. Notice speed breakers. Take note of the vehicles standing nearby while parking your vehicle. If you want to take a taxi, call it to one side of the road and then get into it. Do not try to enter the taxi in the middle of the road.

f) When you are driving a vehicle try to keep at a distance from both vehicles going in front and those who are coming in the back. Be careful, while going through dangerous turns and roads of hilly side. Don't overtake police van, ambulance or fire engine.

g) If any other vehicle is passing by your side, allow it to pass and slow down your vehicle. Be careful of the people walking, animals that are going on the road. Be careful about the children playing on the road.

h) When you are taking out your car from the garage or when you are taking the car in reverse gear, observe carefully the children playing on the ground.

i) You should not drive a car when you are under the influence of liquor. When you are going for a long drive check the car at every 100 to 150 kilometers. During that time, you can drink coffee or tea. You should not drive the vehicle when you are sleepy.

j) When you are going to any institution, follow the rules of the institution. Follow signals and rules when you are going in a lift. Be careful, while going in or coming out of self operated lifts.

k) When you are playing any game, exhibit sportsman spirit. You should not get excited under any circumstances and quarrel. Always keep a first aid box on the play ground.

Safety measures in agriculture

Villagers have no knowledge of facilities available for taking safety measure during their agricultural operations. Even the accidents are generally minor, they may prove fatal because of nonavailability of medical aid and also due to lack of knowledge about safety measures. In a village when people quarrel, they use stones, lathis, pistols and other weapons. So, to avoid such quarrels, the people should be patient. Falling from a tree or a branch of tree falling on a person sleeping under the tree is very common. He may fall from roofs of huts built on the fields. Accident, while using a spade for bringing the side upside is common. Falling from the horse back, bullock cart, tractor or trolley is a common occurrence in villages. Snake bites, scorpion bite etc. are also very common. Electric shock is common while starting or putting off the electric water pump. The villagers should be careful to avoid sunstroke and tiredness and high fever. Due to inhalation of insecticides, there can be severe food poisoning. Loaded bullock carts should not be left on the road because it may cause accidents or quarrels.

Safety measures in industries

Accidents are very common in big factories. These may be due to negligence of the safety measures and the guidelines issued for the prevention of a accidents.

The switches to put on and put off the machines should be fitted nearby. The belts should be as small as possible. There should be safety guards around it. When the motors are working, these guards should be fixed in proper position. The workers in the factory should use plastic shields or transparent shields to protect themselves from dust, excessive heat etc. They should protect the eyes also. The machines used in industries should be run on recognised voltage. High or low voltage cause danger to life and property.

Before starting work in an Industry, it is necessary to accustom yourself with its discipline of working. Always wear shirts of small sleeves. Do not try to use big instruments to do small works. You must use instruments according to the type of work. Before starting your work on any machine, check whether the machine is in working condition or not. Do not bring your face near a working machine. Have sufficient light in the area of work. After the work is finished, the instruments should be cleaned and kept in proper places. Apply grease or oil to the machines for their smooth working. Electrical instruments should be kept away from the children. The Petro Chemical Industries should be properly designed. There should be a separate Fire Extinguishing Unit in the Factory to prevent fire accidents. In cotton and textile industries cotton knots should be collected and divided and kept in small units in the godowns. It is better to fit fire detectors in the factory. In textile industry, acid soda is used to extinguish the fire. Carbon dioxide is generally used to extinguish the fire of electrical equipments.

Safety measures in Hospitals

Minor accidents like falling from the wheel chair, getting wrong medicine etc. Major accidents like fire or explosion may also take place.

So, all workers in the hospital should be careful against such risk. Fire in hospitals is, mainly, due to smoking carelessly in bed, faulty electrical equipments etc. So, in hospitals smoking should be prohibited by hanging board with a warning "No smoking". Faulty equipments should immediately be repaired. Inflammable things should be thrown in a safe place. Electrical machines, anaesthetic gases etc. may cause fire in operation theatres. It may also be due to static electricity and hence the nurses and other staff working in operation theatres, should not wear nylon clothes.

In the hospital, there should be sufficient supply of water and chemical machines to extinguish the fire. When fire breaks out, first inform the incharge officer. Build the courage of the patients to face any eventuality. The workers and patients who can walk, may be asked to close the windows and doors. Electrical equipments and oxygen cylinders should be closed at once. All exit doors should be kept clean. Wet blankets may be placed below the closed doors to keep the wards free from smoke. Patients should be taken away from the fire. Help the hospital staff in controlling and extinguishing the fire.

Falling from bed is one common accident in the hospital. Slipping and falling on very smooth floor is also very common. Do not allow the patients until the floor is dry. Be careful, while carrying patients on stretchers. Due to the carelessness of nurses, patients get burnt with hot water bottle. So, before filling the hot water bottle, its temperature should be checked. The patients should not be allowed to touch electric equipments with wet hands. There may be mistakes in giving medicine by nurses, compounders or doctors. Poisonous medicines should be kept locked in the almirah. Mentally ill patients try to jump out of the window. Nurses should be alert to prevent such an eventuality. Broken instruments should be kept out of reach for the patients.

The workers in the hospitals should be trained to follow safety measures. Children should be looked after with care. Dangerous things like pin, match box etc. should be kept away from children. They should not be allowed to keep small things in the mouth. You should not force children to eat and do not leave them alone when they are eating. There should be a helper to hold the child lightly while giving injection. You should not inject the child when you are alone. Small toys should be removed when the child is sleeping in a cradle.

BURNS AND SCALDS

Causes

1. Burns are injuries that result from dry heat, like fire, flame, a piece of hot metal, or the sun, contact with wire carrying high tension electric current or by lightning or friction. Scalds are caused by moist heat due to boiling water, steam oil, hot tar etc.,

2. Chemical burns are caused by strong acids or by strong alkalies.

3. A nuclear burn is caused by the instantaneous flash of intense heat given off by a nuclear explosion. It is capable of causing superficial burns on the exposed skin of persons several miles away.

First aid treatment for critical burns

Immediate attention that is required in critical burns are as follows:

1. Keep the casualty quiet and reassure him.

2. Wrap him up in clean cloth

3. Do not remove adhering particles of charred clothing.

4. Cover burnt area with sterile or clean dressing and bandage. In case of burns covering a large part of the body, it is sufficient to cover the area with a clean sheet or towel.

5. Keep him warm but do not overheat him.

6. If the hands are involved, keep them above the level of the victims heart.

7. Keep burnt feet or legs elevated.

8. If victims face is burnt, sit up or prop him up and keep under continuous observation for breathing difficulty.

9. Do not immerse the extensive burnt area or apply ice water over it because cold may intensify the shock reaction. However, cold pack may be applied to the face or to the hands or feet.

10. Shift the casualty to the nearest hospital if he is fit to be moved.

11. If you cannot take him to a hospital, wait for the doctor to arrive.

12. Do not open blisters.

13. Keep him wrapped up in clean cloth.

14. Treat for shock.

15. Remove quickly from the body anything of a constricting nature like rings, bangles, belt and boots. If this is not done early, it would be difficult to remove them later as the limb begin to swell.

16. If medical help or trained ambulance personal cannot reach the scene for an hour or more and the victim is conscious and not vomiting, give him a weak solution of salt and soda at home and enroute - one level tea spoonful of salt and half level teaspoonful of salt and half level teaspoonful of baking soda to each pint of water neither hot nor cold. Allow the casualty to sip slowly, give about 4 ounces to an adult over a period of 14 minutes, two ounces to a child between 1 and

12 years of age about one ounce to an infant under one year of age. Discontinue fluid if vomiting occurs. Do not apply ointment or any form of grease or other home remedies.

Classification of burns

On the basis of area : Burns are classified on the basis of area by the **RULE OF NINE**. Any burn of over 30% irrespective of deep degree should be hospitalized as priority.

Burns larger than 2.5 cm (1") square require medical attention.

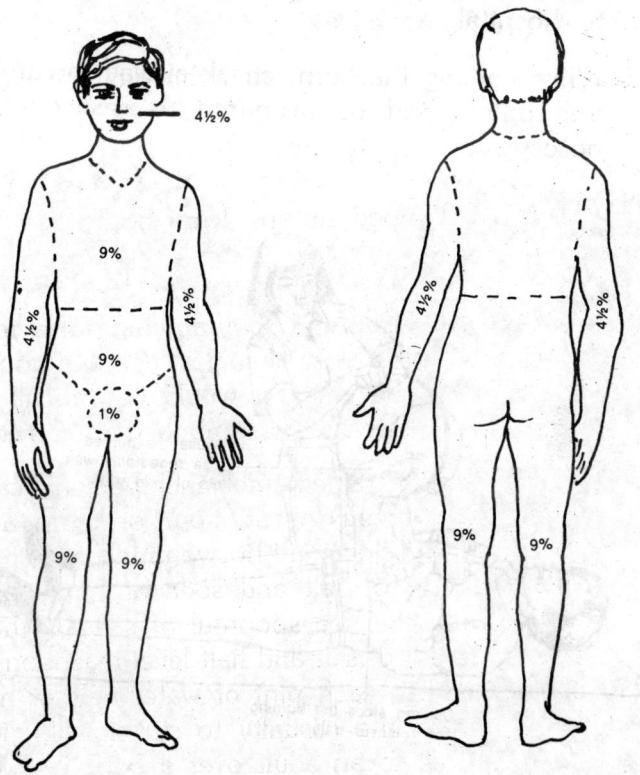

Figure 3. Showing areas divided for calculation of burns

Severe Burns and ·Scalds

Depth, extent, and, possibly, circumstances will swiftly alert you to a burn's severity. The priority is to cool the injury; the longer the burning is allowed to go unchecked, the more severely the casualty will be injured. Follow the ABC of resuscitation only once cooling is under way. Remember, too, that all severe burns carry with them danger of shock.

1. Lay the casualty down, if possible protecting the burned area from contact with the ground.

2. Douse the burn with copious amounts of cold liquid. Thorough cooling may take 10 minutes or more, but this must not delay the casualty's removal to hospital.

3. While cooling the burn, check airway, breathing, and pulse, and be prepared to resuscitate if necessary.

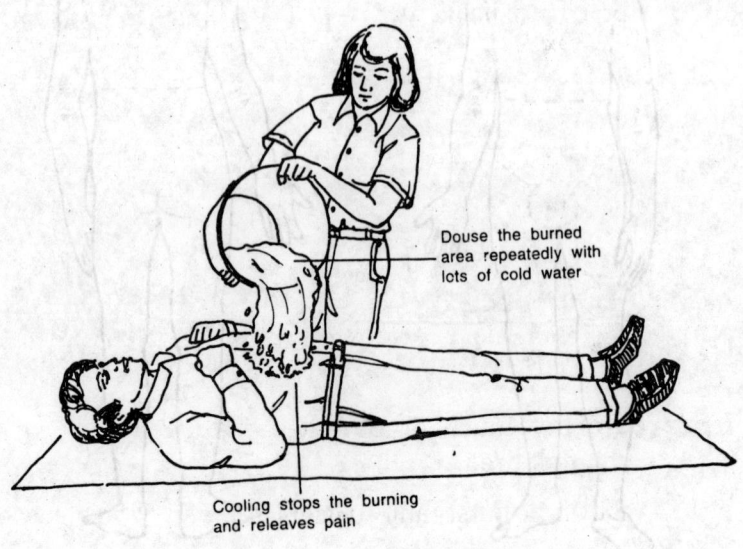

Douse the burned area repeatedly with lots of cold water

Cooling stops the burning and releaves pain

Figure. 4

26

4. Gently remove any rings, watches, belts, shoes, or smouldering clothing from the injured area, before it begins to swell. Carefully remove burned clothing unless it is sticking to the burn.

5. Cover the injury with a sterile burns sheet or other suitable material. (Burns to the face do not need to be covered. Keep cooling them with water to relieve the pain.)

6. Ensure that an ambulance is on its way. While waiting, treat the casualty for shock. Monitor and record breathing and pulse, and be prepared to resuscitate if necessary.

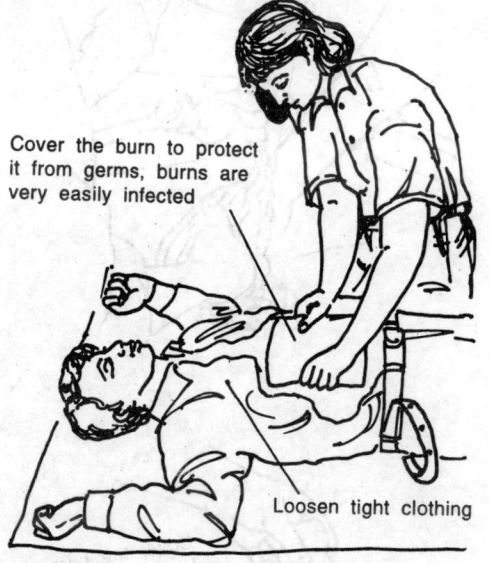

Cover the burn to protect it from germs, burns are very easily infected

Figure. 5

Loosen tight clothing

Note : Do not touch or otherwise interfere with the injured area.

Do not burst any blisters.

Do not apply lotions, ointment or fat to the injury.

Minor burns and scalds

Domestic accidents are the most common cause of minor burns and scalds. Prompt first aid will usually enable them to heal naturally and well, but if you are in any doubt as to the severity of the injury, seek a doctor's advice.

1. Flood the injured part with cold water for about 10 minutes to stop the burning and relieve the pain. If water is unavailable, any cold, harmless liquid, such as milk or canned drinks. will do.

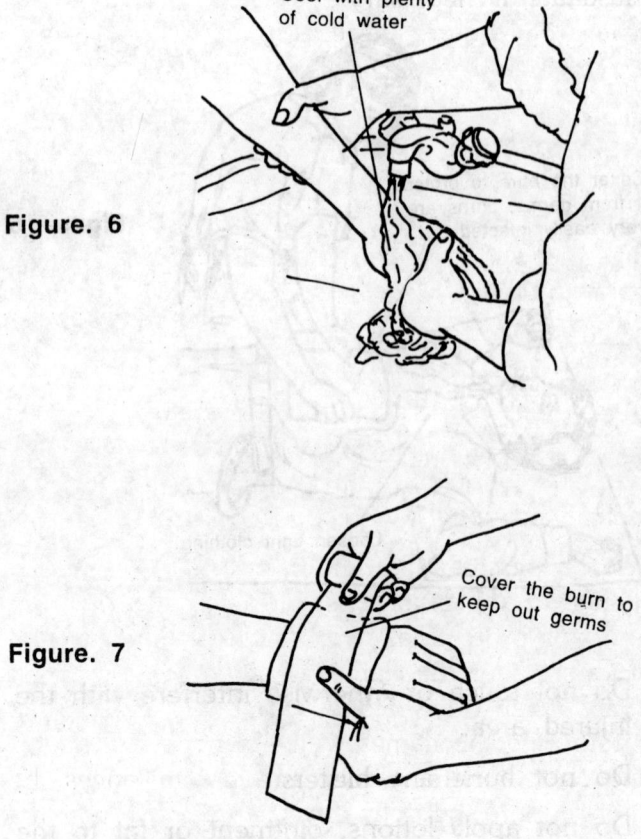

Cool with plenty of cold water

Figure. 6

Cover the burn to keep out germs

Figure. 7

2. Gently remove any jewellery, watches, or constricting clothing from the injured area before it begins to swell.

3. Cover the area with a sterile dressing, or any clean, non-fluffy material. A polythene bag or kitchen film makes a good temporary covering.

The effects of both burns and scalds are the same. The skin may be reddened or blister formed or destruction of the skin, or the deeper tissues.

There will be severe pain. There is immediate danger from shock which may be severe and made worse by the intense pain and by loss of plasma into the burnt area. Later, there is danger from septic infection.

The areas of burns and scalds, including the clothing involved are all intents and purposes sterile for a short period and try your best to keep them so, until medical aid is available. Always use prepared dry sterile dressings and great care must be taken in handling and applying them.

The dangers of a burn increase with its surface area (even if it is only superficial) and if one third or more of the skin area is involved, the patient may become dangerously ill. In small children and infants, even small burns should be considered as serious injuries and medical aid sought without delay.

When a person's clothing catches fire, approach him holding a rug, blanket, coat or table cover, in front of yourself for protection, wrap it round him, lay him flat and so smother the flames. If a person's clothing catches fire when he is alone, he should roll on the floor, smothering the flames with the nearest available wrap and call for help. Under any circumstances, he should not run into the open air. The use of fire guards will prevent many calamities in the home.

29

General rules for the treatment of burns and scalds

1. Do not handle the affected area more than is necessary. Keep your hands clean by thoroughly washing them.

2. Avoid applying lotions of any kind.

3. Do not remove burned clothing and do not break blisters.

4. If possible, cover the area (including burned clothing) with a prepared dry sterile dressing. Otherwise clean lint freshly laundered linen or some similar material can be used.

5. Bandage firmly except when blisters are present. If blisters are present, bandage lightly.

6. Immobilise the affected area by proper means.

7. Treat for shock.

   a) In a major case, remove the patient to the hospital as quickly as possible. The patient may require an anaesthetic, so that, nothing should ordinarily be given by the mouth. If medical aid is delayed beyond four hours, give drinks of water to which salt has been added in the proportion of half a teaspoon to two tumblers, approximately 1/2 a teaspoon of bicarbonate of soda may be added.

   b) In a minor case give large quantities of warm fluids, preferably, weak tea sweetened with sugar.

When the face is burnt

1. Cut from a piece of clean lint, a dressing in the shape of a mask with a hole for breathing.

2. Maintain in position by a bandage like that of fractured jaw.

Treatments of burns caused by corrosive chemicals

1. When the corrosive is an acid :-

    a) Flood the part thoroughly with water.

    b) Bathe the part freely with some alkaline solution, such as, two teaspoons of baking soda (bicarbonate of soda) or washing soda, carbonate of soda) in one pint of warm water.

    c) Apply general rules for treatment of burns. Remove contaminated clothing as quickly as possible to avoid further injury. Take reasonable precautions against burning yourself with contaminated clothing.

2. When the corrosive is an alkali:-

    a) If the burn is caused by quick lime, brush off any that may remain on the part.

    b) Flood the part thoroughly with water.

    c) Bathe part freely with a weak acid solution such as, vinegar or lemon juice, diluted with an equal amount of warm water.

    d) Apply general rules for the treatment of burns. Remove any contaminated clothing at once, taking necessary precautions.

Chemical burns

Certain chemicals may irritate or damage the skin, or be absorbed through the skin, or be absorbed through the skin, causing widespread and sometimes fatal damage within the body. Unlike thermal burns, the signs of chemical burns develop slowly. The principles of first aid are however, the same.

Most strong corrosives are found in industry, though chemical burns can also be caused by domestic agents such as oven cleaners and paint stripper. These injuries are always serious, and may require urgent hospital treatment. It may be helpful to discover and note the name or brand name, of the substance. Ensure your own safety when approaching and treating these injuries; note that some chemicals give off deadly fumes.

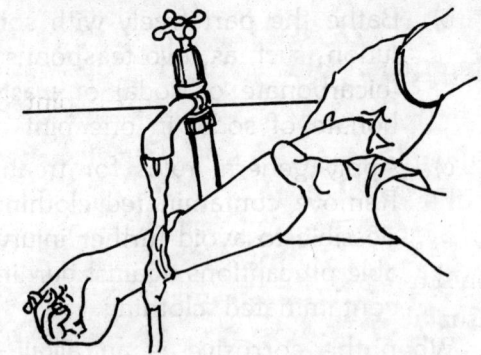

Figure 8

1. Flood the affected area with water to disperse the chemical and stop the burning process. Irrigate for longer than you would for a thermal burn; some chemicals may need 20 minutes.

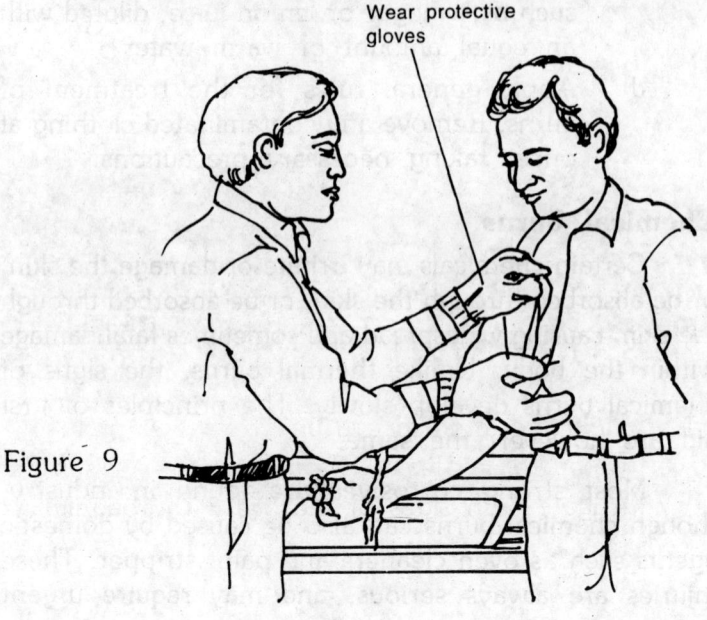

Wear protective gloves

Figure 9

2. Gently remove any contaminated clothing while flooding the injury. Be sure not to contaminate yourself – use protective gloves if available.

3. Take or send the casualty to hospital, keeping a close watch on airway and breathing.

Chemicals Burns to the eye

Splashes of chemicals in the eye can cause serious injury if not treated quickly. They can damage the surface of the eye, resulting in scarring and even blindness. Be especially careful, while irrigating the eye, that contaminated rinsing water does not splash you or the casualty. Wear protective gloves if they are available.

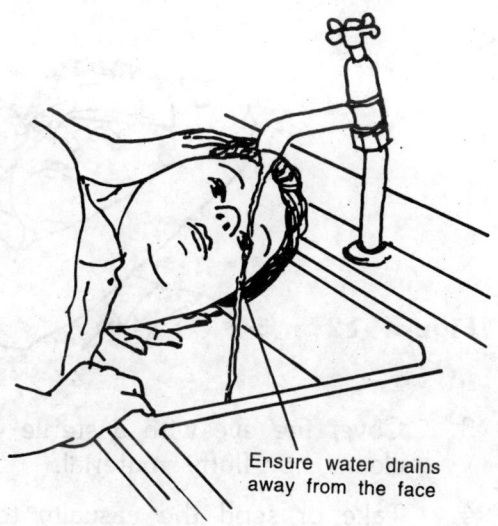

Figure 10

Ensure water drains away from the face

1. Hold the affected eye under gently running cold water for at least 10 minutes. Make sure you irrigate both sides of the eyelid thoroughly. You may find it easier to pour the water from an eye irrigator or a glass.

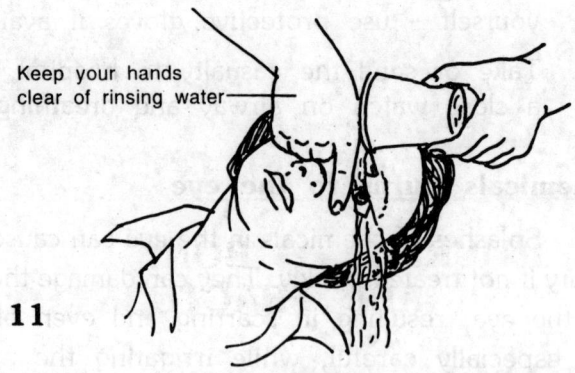

Keep your hands
clear of rinsing water

Figure 11

2. If the eye is shut in a spasm of pain, gently but firmly pull the eyelids open. Be careful that contaminated water does not splash the sound eye.

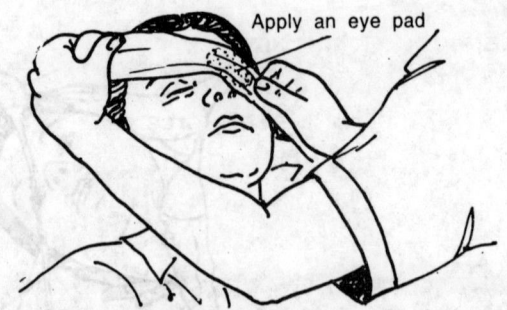

Apply an eye pad

Figure 12

3. Cover the eye with a sterile eye pad or pad of clean, non-fluffy material.

4. Take or send the casualty to hospital.

34

INJURIES TO BONE, JOINTS AND FRACTURES

Bones form the supporting framework of our body. Traffic accidents, falls, assaults and crush injuries, result in injuries to bones. When the bone is partially or completely broken it is called "fracture".

A fracture means that a bone is broken or cracked.

Causes of fracture

1. Direct force: When the bone breaks at the place where force is applied.
2. Indirect force: The bone that breaks is away from the place where force is applied.
3. The force of muscular action.
4. Diseased bone: Bones of old age, break easily with very little force.

Types of fractures

1. **Close or simple fracture:** It is the one in which there is no wound leading down to the broken bone and the bone has not cut through the skin.

2. **Open or compound fractures:** It is the one in which the broken bone is in contact with the outside of air as a result of the injury. In such cases, germs get into the wound including the bone.

3. **Complicated fracture:** When in connection with the fracture, there is injury to some important internal part. A complicated fracture may be either open or closed.

4. **Communited fracture:** When the bone is broken into several pieces.

5. **Depressed fracture:** A fracture of the skull when the broken part is driven inwards by pressing the brain.

6. **Green stick fracture:** This occurs in children when the bone is cracked and bent without breaking completely across. A fracture dislocation may occur when the bone is close to the joint.

7. **Impacted fracture:** Where the broken bones ride over one another.

Signs and symptoms of fracture

1. Pain in the fractured part.

2. Tenderness or discomfort or gentle pressure over the injured spot.

3. Swelling of the area.

4. Dislocation may appear soon after the injury or after a few days.

5. Loss of normal movements of the part injured.

6. Deformity of the limb, normal shape is altered or the limb is shortened.

7. Irregularity, if the broken bone is close under the skin.

8. Unnatural movement and credetes, only a doctor may examine for these signs.

To conform diagnosis compare with the uninjured limb, mark on the clothing or skin may help to locate the fracture. The casualty may have heard the snap of the bone.

First aid treatment of fractures

The aims of first aid are:

1. To prevent further damage
2. To reduce pain and shock
3. To make the patient feel comfortable
4. To get medical aid as soon as possible

The general rules are as follows

1. Treat the fracture on the spot. Do not move the casualty, unless there is danger to life, until the injured part has been immobilised.

2. Handle very gently and avoid all unnecessary movements of the injured part.

3. Steady and support the injured part at once preventing movement which could result in further injury.

4. If it is an open fracture, cut away clothing over the wound, stop bleeding and cover with a dry sterile dressing.

5. Treat for shock, reassuring the casualty.

6. Immobilise the fracture area and the joints above and below the fracture site by means of bandage or splints.

7. Do not attempt too much. Never try to bring the bones to normal position or reduce the fracture. Keep to simple first aid.

Using bandages

1. For simple first aid, it is usually enough to tie a broken arm to the body or the broken, to the good leg.

2. Do not apply a bandage over the site of the fracture.

37

3. Tie bandages firmly enough to prevent movement but not so tightly as to stop the circulation of blood to the part.

4. Always place padding in hollow and between the ankles and knees, so that limbs are comfortable when tied.

5. With the casualty lying, it is best to double the bandage over a splint or similar object and to pass it under the natural hollow, like the neck, knees and ankles. Avoid lifting and jarring the casualty while working the bandages into correct position.

6. Tie the knots on the uninjured side, or on the splint, if one is used.

Using splints

Splints may be required if a long, difficult journey is necessary or if both legs are broken. Splints may be made of any firm material, such as, wood, plastic or metal. The splint should be wide enough to fit well to the limb and long enough to immobilise the joint above and below the fracture. It should be well padded and applied over the clothing.

Splints may be improvised from a piece of wood, card board, folded newspaper or an umbrella or stick. The body itself is used as a splint, as in above.

After fixing splints and bandages, always check that they are firm enough to properly immobilise the part, but not so tight as to prevent the circulation of blood.

Indications for the use of splints

The first aider must use his discretion before using splints. When there is likely to be considerable delay before medical services become available, when the distance to hospital is long, when the patient has to be carried over uneven ground and when the injured limb cannot be satisfactorily supported against a sound part of the body, splints can·be used.

The main object of splinting as a first aid procedure is to prevent a fracture becoming compound or complicated during transport. Splints also provide complete rest to the injured parts and hence, relieve pain and encourage healing. Splints keep the fragments aligned, so that, the bone is restored to its natural shape after healing takes place.

Types of splint

There are several kinds of splints,

1. **Wooden:** Straight pieces of wood of varying lengths and widths, can be used as splints.

2. **Metal:** Splints made of tin and aluminum are commonly in use. Metal splints can be got padded with felt and ready for immediate use.

3. **Kramer's wire splinting:** It is very popular because it can be quickly cut into required length. It is made of a framework of metal which is strengthened by struts placed across it. It is moulded from side to side to fit the natural curvature of the limbs.

4. **Plaster:** Plaster of Paris is used by surgeons in the treatment of fractures. Special splints can easily be made to suit individual needs. First aiders may be asked to help in the application of this method and so, they must have some knowledge of this method. Roller bandages of different widths are used for this purpose. The limb about to be encased, should be protected with stockinette or cotton wool. Then, it is covered with layers of plaster of Paris using roller· bandaging methods. The plaster sets firmly within a few seconds.

Plaster of Paris should never be used by first aiders without medical supervision.

5. **Inflatable splint:** It is a new piece of apparatus. It is gaining popularity rapidly and it may be widely used in first aid and may become an essential piece of equipment to be kept in the ambulance.

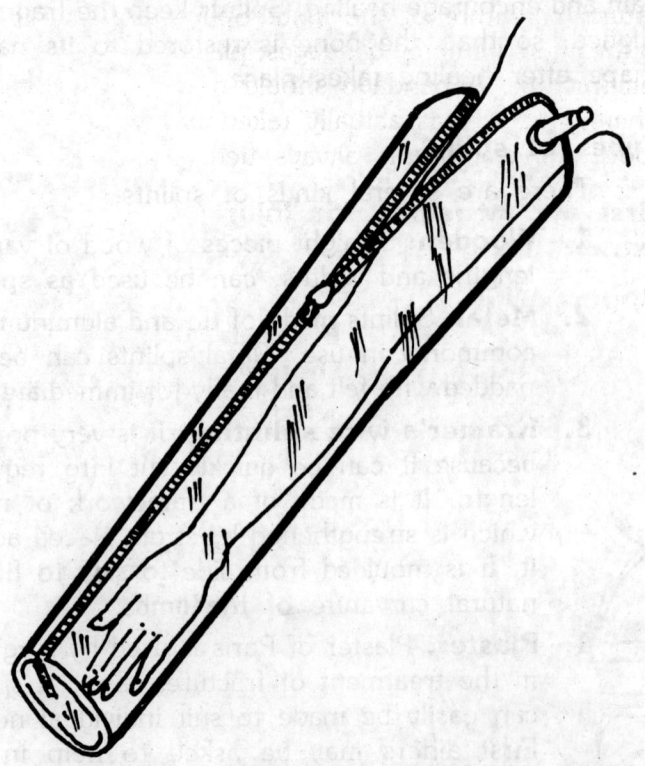

Figure 13. The inflatable splint

There are several varieties of inflatable splint, but in general, those with metal zips, are preferable to those having plastic zips. The leg splint has the zip placed in front. Sometimes, the splint gets partially deflated. The patient does not get the expected satisfaction. So, the users should be given suitable instructions before use.

Application of splints

The splints chosen, should be sufficiently strong and of suitable length and width. The splint should be long enough to keep the joints immediately above and below the fracture at rest. The splint should be covered with cotton wool or tow. This may be secured in position by linen sewn on to the back of the splint. It is desirable to choose a splint which is suitably moulded to fit the natural curvature of the limb. Splints should be fixed to the injured limb by bandages, placed above and below the fracture. A bandage should never encircle a limb where fracture has actually taken place. The bandage above the fracture is always tied.

First aid measures for injuries to upper extremities.

Upper arm

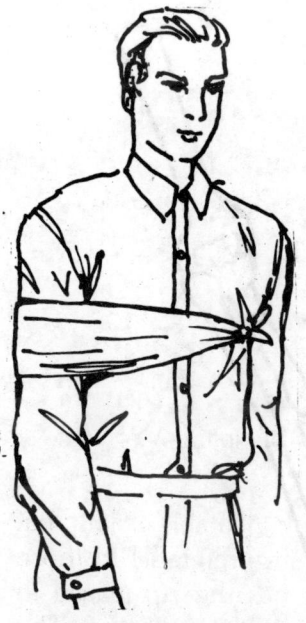

Figure 14. Fracture of the Collar bone

If the fracture is close to shoulder,

1. Place a pad in the axilla.
2. Lightly tie the arm to the chest.
3. Bend the elbow, and, with the hand on the opposite shoulder, apply a collar and cuffsling.

If the fracture is in the Mid Shaft,

1. Place a pad between arm and chest.
2. Tie the upper arm firmly to the chest, one bandage above and the other below the site of fracture.
3. Support the forearm in the sling.

41

If the fracture is near the elbow

1. The elbow can be bent. Tie the arm to the chest and support the forearm in a triangular sling.

2. If the elbow cannot be bent, get the casualty to lie down, and tie the arm to the trunk in extended position.

Forearm

Colles's fracture, near to the wrist, is very common. It is caused by a fall on the outstretched hand. There will be swelling and deformity at the wrist.

Treatment: It is best to use a splint for first aid in forearm fractures. A folded newspaper or magazine will serve well, if it extends from the elbow to the fingers.

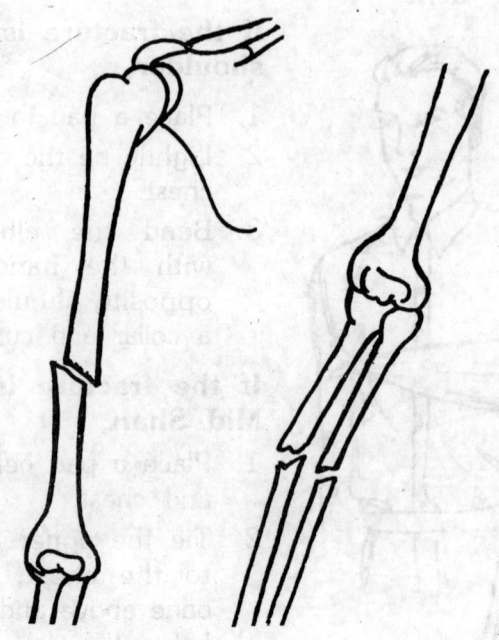

Figure 15. Fracture of the forearm

1. Place the forearm across the chest at right angle with thumb finger uppermost and palm of the hand towards the body.
2. Roll the folded newspaper or magazine around the forearm.
3. Apply one bandage above the fracture and a second, as a figure of eight, around the wrist and hand.
4. Support the arm in a sling with fingers, slightly higher than the elbow.
5. Watch the fingers for signs of interference with the blood circulation, in which case, loosen the bandage slightly.

First aid measures for injuries to lower extremities

Femur: This bone could break at any place. Fracture of the neck of the femur is common in elderly people. Fracture of the femur are always serious.

Signs and Symptoms
1. Pain, swelling and shock.
2. Shortening of limb.
3. The foot on the injured side, lies turned to the outside.

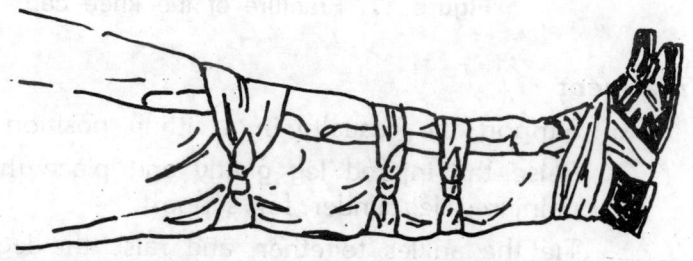

Figure 16. Fracture of lower limbs (leg)

Treatment

1. Treat for shock.
2. Pad between the legs and brings the good leg along side the injured one.
3. Tie together the knees, ankles, hips, above and below the fracture.
4. If there is a long and difficult journey to the hospital, two well padded splints should be applied. One, between the legs, the other, on the outside extending from axilla to the foot. Secure the splints with bandages around the chest, pelvis, knees, above and below the fracture, lower legs, a figure of eight around the ankles and knee.

Patella: Fracture of the patella may occur due to direct force, but is more often, due to muscular action.

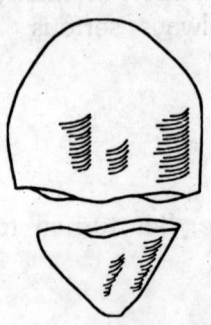

Signs and symptoms

1. The limb is helpless
2. There is much swelling
3. The gap may be felt between the two bits of bone.

Figure 17. Fracture of the knee cap

Treatment

1. Support the casualty in a sitting position.
2. Raise the injured leg gently and place the uninjured leg under for support.

   Tie the ankles together, and raise the legs on a box. The legs may be tied together by means of a narrow bandage above the knee in a figure of eight bandage.

44

3. If a splint is available, apply it to the base of the limb, it should reach from the buttock to beyond the heel, pad under the ankle, and secure the splint to the limb by bandages round the thigh, ankle and figure of eight, above and below the knee.

Lower leg: The tibia only, or both and tibula may be broken. All the signs of fracture are seen in these cases. If the tibia only is much swelling around, the ankle fracture of ankle bones also, should be suspected.

Treatment

Treat as for femur fracture, but without the long splint.

Foot and Toes

This fracture is caused by direct force, like a crush injury.

Treatment

1. Remove footwear and treat wounds.

2. Raise and support the foot

3. Apply a padded splint to the sole of the foot.

4. Secure the splint with a figure of eight bandage. Start with the centre of broad bandage on the splints, cross-the ends over the instep and carry them to the back of the ankle and again cross once more, to bring them to the front of the ankle. Cross once more to bring the ends to the foot, cross and tie it off over the centre of the splint.

5. Transport the casualty by stretcher with the foot raised.

First aid measure for skull injuries

A direct blow or fall on the head, may cause fracture of the upper part of the skull, is often a depressed fracture.

A fall on the feet or buttocks or a blow to the lower jaw may cause fracture of the base of the skull when blood or brain fluid may be seen coming from the ear or nose.

Fracture of the skull, may cause unconsciousness immediately or coming later.

Treatment

1. If breathing is not noisy, lay the casualty on his back with head and shoulder slightly raised.

2. If breathing is noisy, place the casualty into the recovery position with head to one side. If there is bleeding from the ear, turn the head so that, the bleeding side is down.

3. Do not try to rouse the casualty. Keep him quiet and undisturbed.

4. Keep the head still during transport, using sand bags or pads.

5. Treat for shock and refer immediately.

Rib Injuries

Ribs may be broken by direct force, or indirectly by a crush injury. There is danger that the broken ribs may be driven inwardly causing injury to the lungs.

Signs and Symptoms

1. Pain that is made worse by coughing or deep breathing.

2. The casualty taken short, shallow breaths, so that, the ribs do not move and increase the pain.

3. If the lung is injured, blood may be coughed up.

4. If there is an open wound in the chest, air is sucked in and blows out as the casualty breaths. This is a serious complication.

Treatment

1. Uncomplicated fracture of the ribs

   a) Apply two broad bandages to the area of pain. The upper bandage should overlap the lower one by half its width. Tie them lightly first after the casualty has breathed out, with knotsnear the front on the uninjured side.

   b) Support the arm to the injured side in a sling.

2. Complicated fracture of the ribs:-

   a) If there is a sucking wound, cover it with a dry dressing pad bandage firmly. In other cases, do not apply bandages.

   b) Support the casualty with head and shoulders raised and turned towards the injured side, transport carefully in the position on a stretcher.

   c) A sling may be applied to the arm on the injured side.

Injuries to pelvis

Fracture of the pelvis, usually, occurs due to direct force such as, in the crush accident. The pelvic organs, especially, the bladder or urethra may be injured.

Signs and Symptoms

1. Pain in the hips when they are pressed together.

2. The casualty is unable to stand, nor to move the legs without pain.

3. There may be an urge to pass urine, but he is unable to do so or finds it difficult.

4. There may be internal bleeding.

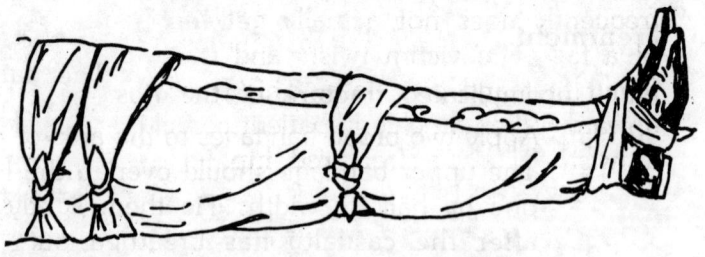

Figure 18. Treatment of fractured pelvis

Treatment

1. Lay the casualty in the most comfortable position. If he wants to stand up his knees, support them with folded clothing or pillow.

2. Ask him to avoid passing urine.

3. If a hospital is near, transport him on a stretcher without bandaging.

4. If the journey is long and on rough roads, apply pads between the knees and ankles, then tie two overlapping broad bandages or a towel around the pelvis. Bandages should be tied on the uninjured side.

5. Tie the knees together, with a broad bandage.

6. Tie a figure of eight bandage around the ankles and feet.

48

Fracture of femur

Fracture of neck of femur

This fracture occurs in an elderly patient as a result of fall. The elderly osteoporotic bone is usually fractured as a result of sudden twisting. The victim frequently does not actually get the fracture because of a fall. The victim twists and fractures the neck of femur first and then falls. This fracture runs obliquely upward. When an elderly patient complains of pain after a twist or fall, a fractured hip is usually suspected.

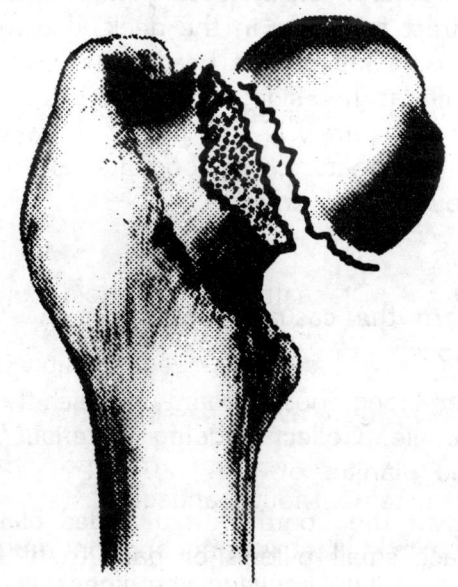

Figure 19. Fracture of neck of femur

Signs and symptoms

1. Painful hip and some degree of shock.
2. Shortening and slight external rotation of the neck.
3. Failure to recognise, leads to displacement of femoral neck.

Treatment

1. Treat for shock.

2. Protect the hip by using crutches until the pain subsides and X-rays can be obtained.

3. Protect the hip by padding, and immobilise the part.

4. The patient should be transported to a hospital in a lying position for further treatment.

First aid measures for spinal injuries

Spinal fracture, usually, occurs either in the lumbar region by direct force, or in the neck, due to indirect force, such as, a fall on the head. The casualty complains of pain at the side. The spinal cord may be damaged causing paralysis and loss of sensation below the side of the fracture. By good first aid treatment, paralysis may be prevented.

Treatment

1. Warn the casualty not to move. Treat for shock.

2. Get a long enough board on which the casualty can lie. Collect padding material, bandages and blanket or rug.

3. Cover the board with a folded blanket and place small pillows or pads to fit the neck and middle of the back.

4. Atleast four helpers are needed to get the casualty lying on the board. First place padding between legs. Tie together the ankles and feet with figure of eight bandage, and to his knees together.

5. When all are ready, the helper must carry together and be very careful not to bend or

twist the spine as they either roll the casualty or lift him to get him on the prepared board. One should hold the head firmly and keep the neck straight. Another hold the legs near the ankles, while other keep the shoulder and hips steady and in line.

6. Tie the casualty to the board to prevent movement during transport.

7. If there is a neck injury, do not use a pillow under the neck, but place bags of sand or firm pads on each side of the bed to keep from moving.

8. Take the casualty to hospital or health centre, as soon as possible.

Crush injuries

In major accidents, people may be caught under machinery, masonry and beams and may be crush for several hours, when released, the casualty may complain only of numbness in the injured parts. Injuries may be seen with swelling and general condition, quite good.

After sometime, there may be serious reaction, toxic substances from crushed cells, pour into the blood stream causing severe shock, kidney failure may also occur.

Treatment

1. Get casualty released and take to hospital, as quickly as possible.

2. If shifting is delayed and the casualty is conscious, give him tender coconut or water frequently.

3. When relaxed, raise the injury part and leave it uncovered for observation. Allow the circulation to return gradually. Never apply heat.

51

Multiple fractures

When the bone is broken into several pieces, it occurs in the knee or patella. It is caused by a direct blow to the patella, such as, when the knee strikes the dash board in a car accident.

Signs and symptoms

1. Swelling is present
2. The patient will have severe pain
3. Deformity

Management

1. Lay the casualty flat with head and shoulders raised.

   The injured limb should be raised to an easy position. This will relax the thigh muscles which pull the upper half of the broken bone upwards.

2. Tie to sound limb from thigh to below knee with padding between knees.

3. Apply a padded splint from the buttocks to beyond the heel. The ankle should be raised from the splint by pads.

   a) Apply a broad bandage around the upper part of the thigh.

   b) Apply a narrow figure of eight bandage around the ankle and foot.

   c) Place a narrow bandage with its center on the upper fractured piece, cross it behind the knees and bring it up, over the lower fractured bit and tie it off.

4. During transport also, the limb should be kept raised on a box, blanket or similar material.

___

ROAD ACCIDENTS, WOUNDS WITH BLEEDING & HAEMORRHAGE

Road accidents

Road accidents range from a fall from bicycle to a major accident with many casualties. Often the accident site will present serious risks to safety large because of oncoming traffic. It is essential to make the area safe to protect yourself, the casualty and other pedestrians.

i) Make the accident site safe.

ii) First ensure your own safety.

iii) Do not run across a busy motorway to reach the other side.

iv) Switch off the vehicle.

v) Check the casualties.

If there is a neck injury, support the casualty's head and neck with your hands.

i) Attend to any life threatening injuries if possible. Observe the casualty continuously until the expert help arrives.

ii)   If a casualty is trapped under a vehicle try to find help to lift or move the vehicle and if absolutely necessary, drag the casualty clear.

Wounds and bleeding

Any abdominal break in the skin on body surfaces is known as a wound. Most wounds are open – with a break in the skin through which blood and other fluid may be lost from the body, and germs may enter and cause infection. A closed wound allows blood to escape from the circulatory system, but not the body – the condition known as internal bleeding.

In cases of wounds and bleeding the first-aider should:

1.   Control blood loss by applying pressure over the wound and raising the injured part.

2.   Take steps to minimise shock, which may be caused by extensive blood loss.

3.   Protect the wound from infection, and promote natural healing, by covering it with a dressing.

4.   Since germs can be present in body fluids, at all times pay attention to hygiene, both to protect the casualty and yourself.

When any tissue of the body e.g. skin, muscle, bone etc. is torn or cut by injury, a wound is caused. There will be bleeding from the injured part and it also forms an opening through which germs can get into the body. The depth of a wound is often, more important than its area, small deep wound caused by knives, bullets etc. are often, the more dangerous.

Principles of wound care

The principles of wound care are as follows:-

1.   To stop the bleeding
2.   To prevent infection

54

Immediate care in wound and bleeding

1. Stop bleeding: Apply direct pressure to the wound with a sterile dressing or a clean hand kerchief. If necessary, press on the ARTERIAL pressure point.

2. Handle the injured part as gently as possible.

3. If the wound is in a limb and there are no broken bones, raise the limb. This will lessen the bleeding.

4. Wash your hands thoroughly.

5. Remove any foreign objects like glass, stones etc. if you can easily get at them. This should not open up the wound again, which will cause more bleeding. Do not disturb any blood clot already formed.

6. Place a clean dressing over the wound and bandage firmly.

7. Get a doctor.

If you cannot get a doctor or nurse, reach him to one within 6-8 hours.

HAEMORRHAGE

Haemorrhage is a common cause of death in accidents. It is caused by the rupture of blood vessels due to severity of the injury.

Types of bleeding

Bleeding may occur from a) arteries, b) veins or c) capillaries, or from a combinations of the three.

a) Bleeding from Arteries:-

The blood comes out in jets, because, it corresponds to the beats of the heart in action. The blood will be bright red. This kind of bleeding may cause death very quickly.

b) Bleeding from veins: Blood flows out in a continuous stream and is dark red in colour.

c) Bleeding from capillaries: Blood oozes out slowly. If it is on the surface of the body, it is not at all serious.

Control of bleeding

a) Minor Bleeding: Minor bleeding is usual at work and play. It results from injured capillaries. There is no need to get frightened. The bleeding will stop by itself or by firm pressure and bandaging.

b) Major bleeding: Major bleeding is the result of an injury to a large blood vessel or when persons suffer from blood diseases.

Pressure points to stop bleeding

The second method of indirect stopping of haemorrhage is the use of pressure points. This is adopted when direct pressure becomes a failure. There are quite a large number of pressure points which must be remembered by the first aider, so that, he can use the method in emergencies. Pressure point is an area where an artery along its course, can be pressed against an underlying bone, so as to prevent the flow of blood beyond that point. Generally, you can feel pulsations of such points.

1. Carotid pressure point

i) Two in number, one on either side. These arteries arise from the aorta and pass up the neck on either side of the trachea or windpipe to supply blood to the head area.

ii) Pressure is applied by the thumb, placed in the hollow beneath the ice box and the prominent sternomastoid muscle nearby. It is pressed against the vertebral column behind it.

iii) In cut throat cases, in addition to the digital pressure to be applied as described at above, the first aider has to apply digital pressure on the jugular vein above the wound from which blood will be oozing out because this vein is also usually injured along with the artery in these cases. In the event of bleeding not stopping, even then, digital pressure has to be applied below the wound also. Cover the wound, treat for shock and take the casualty immediately to a doctor. The pressure on the bleeding points should be continued till the doctor tells you to remove pressure.

2. **Subclavian pressure point**

   i) As the name indicates, these (two) arteries run behind the clavicles on either side.

   ii) These are branches of the aorta, which run from behind the inner end of the clavicle, across the first ribs on to the armpits.

   iii) Pressure is applied by pressing one thumb on top of the other in the hollow above and behind the middle of the collar bone, so that, the artery is pressed against the first rib.

   iv) Before applying pressure, bare the neck and upper part of the chest. Depress the shoulders and bend his head to the injured side. These make it easy to see the area and get the muscles relaxed, making the work easy.

3. **Facial pressure point**

   i) The palm is placed across the upper part of the neck in such a way that the thumb is on the lower position of the lower jaw and the fingers on the back of the head and neck.

   ii) Pressure is applied on the artery at a point which is the junction between the mid third and posterior line of the lower jaw.

4. Temporal pressure point

i) The palm is placed, so that, the thumb is in a line with upper margin of the ear and the rest of palm over the back of the head.

ii) Pressure is applied above an inch in front of the upper part of the ear backwards against the temporal bone. The temporal artery runs at this place before it gives of branches.

5. Brachial pressure point

i) The brachial arteries run along the inner border of the bicep and branches out to supply the upper limb.

ii) Apply pressure on the middle third of the arm, by passing your fingers under the area.

iii) It is compressed against the humerus.

6. Radial or Ulnar pressure point

i) As these names indicate, these lower parts of the radial ulnar arteries pass over the wrist into the palm to form the palm or arch.

ii) Each of them can be compressed by pressing the thumb against the bone, just above the wrists.

7. Palmar arch pressure point

i) As noted above, the arch is formed by anastamosis of the terminal points of the radial and nar arteries, beyond the middle of the palm.

ii) Pressure is applied by single thumb which is placed flat across, whilst the rest of the palm and fingers are on the back of the injured palm.

8. Femoral pressure point

i) Femoral arteries are of the thighs. They are a continuation of the abdominal aorta, they help to supply the lower limbs with blood.

ii) The artery enters the thigh, above the midway in the groinfold and runs a little inwards, upto the upper two thirds of the thigh and then passes to the back of the knee.

iii) To apply pressure, bend the keens slightly, grasp the thigh with both hands, so that, each of the thumbs is at about the centre of the groin. Place the left thumb over the right and apply pressure directly backwards, against the pelvic bone.

Bleeding from special regions and cavities

NOSE

1. Habitual bleeding during day is common among youngsters. This is not caused by any injury.

2. Adults may bleed from the front portion of the nostril due to minor injury, like, blowing the nose, or picking out crusts.

3. High blood pressure may also cause bleeding through the nose.

Management

1. Bleeding, usually, stops in 10 to 15 minutes.

2. Seat the casualty with the head slightly bent forwards.

3. Ask him to breathe through the mouth. •

4. Loosen clothing at neck.

5. Pinch' the soft part of the nostrils together firmly.

6. Apply a cold compress to the nose for 10 minutes.

7. Ask patient not to blow his nose for some hours.

8. Advise him to see the doctor.

STOMACH

Stomach haemorrhage is, usually, due to an ulcer. The blood is vomited, It may be in red clots, or be partly digested and look like coffee grounds. The casualty complains of abdominal pain.

Management

1. Reassure and keep him lying flat and quite.

2. Give nothing by mouth

3. Take him to a doctor, urgently

LUNGS

Bleeding from the lungs is also called haemoptysis. Blood is coughed up, bright red and frothy.

Management

1. Reassure the casualty and keep him quiet.

2. Lay him down, inclined to the affected side with head and shoulders raised and supported.

3. Let him cough but without effort.

4. Transport urgently, to hospital in the same position.

GUMS

After teeth extraction, bleeding from teeth socket may occur immediately or after a few hours.

Management

1. Rinse mouth with water or saline.

2. Place a thick cotton wool ball in the socket and ask him to bite on it.

3. Send the patient to dentist or a doctor.

Internal bleeding

The aim of first aid is to prevent the conditions from altering worse.

1. Lay the casualty down with the head low. Raise his legs by the use of pillows etc.

2. Keep him calm and relaxed. Reassure him, do not allow him to move.

3. Keep up the body heat with thin blankets, rugs or coats.

4. Do not give anything to eat or drink because he may have to be given anesthesia later.

5. Do not apply hot water bottles or ice bags to chest or abdomen. This might only make things worse.

6. Take him to a hospital as quickly as possible, transport gently.

BOWEL

The large intestines is about 1 meters long and six centimeters in diameter. It contains no digestive glands but it can absorb water, salts and some other substances. The water is absorbed from the waste material, received from the small intestine and it will become more solid which will be the stool or faeces. Faeces are moved on, by slow peristalsis and collect in the last part of the large intestine called the rectum which lies in the back of the pelvis. The rectum leads to the anal canal., 4 cm long, with the sphincter muscle and an opening on the skin, called anus. If the blood is seen in the lower bowel or anus, find out the cause.

1. Reassure him
2. Advise him to take plenty of oral fluids to prevent constipation.
3. Advise him to take fruits, green leaf vegetables.
4. Apply little cold pack
5. Refer the case to the doctor

EAR

This is due to the injury to the head, the blood and C.S.F.(Cerebro Spinal Fluid) may flow out of the ear.

Management

1. Fix a dressing to the ear.
2. Lay the casualty on the floor with the head tilted to the affected side.
3. Keep the head in the same position, even while transporting to the hospital.
4. Transport the patient immediately to the hospital without delay.

KIDNEY

The Kidney's are two beans shaped organs, situated behind the peritoneum, at the back of the abdomen in the region of the last ribs. On either side of the vertebral column, each kidney lies in a bed of fat which has got an outer fibrous coat called capsule for its protection. The kidney substances are made up of twisted tubes called nephrons. Each nephron has a cup shaped end in which the lopes of capillaries bringing blood, containing water and waste products to be excreted. This material passed from the blood into the nephrons and urine is formed. When there is any closed abdominal injury, the blood may flow into the abdomen, as a result of injury, to the kidney may be one of the cause of bleeding. Get the correct history of accidents.

Signs and symptoms

1. Pain may be present in the region of the last ribs and the pain may increase during respiration.

2. Swelling will be present and shock and its symptoms will be present, like, pallor, cold and clammy skin. Rapid pulse, shallow breathing, nausea, vomiting etc.

Management

1. Control external bleeding, if there is anything. Treat other wounds and injuries, like fracture, bruise etc.

2. Nothing should be given by mouth

3. Pulse respiration should be recorded every half an hour.

4. Loosen the clothes

5. Reassure the patient

6. Transport him quickly to a hospital, send for the medical aid.

WOUNDS

Wounds can be classified as follows:

1. **Abrasion (Scratches, grazes & pressure marks):** It is a superficial injury, involving only the outer layers of the skin. It may be caused by friction with a rough object.

2. **Bruise (Contusions):** It is caused by blunt force i.e, stick, stone or fist. There is infiltration of blood into the tissues. There may be rupture of vessels which makes it appear red.

3. **Lacerated wound:** Skin and under lying tissues are torn, as a result of blunt force. They have irregular torn edges and bleed less. These wounds are caused by industrial accidents, falling over of houses, roofs or walls etc.

4. **Incised wounds:** It is an injury caused by a weapon with a sharp cutting edge, like, knife, razor etc. The edges of the wound are clean cut. All the tissues are clearly cut including blood vessels. Hence, they bleed much.

5. **Punctured wound:** It is an injury caused by a pointed weapon which is driven in, through the skin. The vital organs of the body may also be affected.

FIRES

In case of fire rapid, clear thinking is vital. Fire spreads very quickly, so warn any people at risk and alert the fire service immediately.

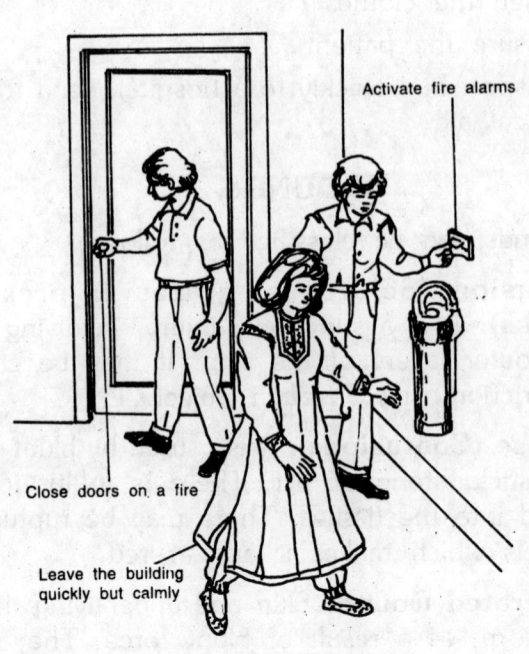

Activate fire alarms

Close doors on a fire

Leave the building quickly but calmly

Figure 20

Without putting yourself at risk, do your best to help everyone if fire occurs in a building or house. Shut the doors behind you look for the notices giving the location. of the fire exits and assembly points. Familiarize yourself with guidelines at your work place.

Dealing with a fire·

A fire needs three components to start it and keep it going. They are ignition (an electric spark or naked flame), a source of fuel such as petrol, wood, or fabrics, and oxygen (air). Remove any one of these and you break this triangle of fire. For example, switch off electricity, remove combustible materials and shut door on a fire, smoother flames with an impervious substance such as blanket or wood.

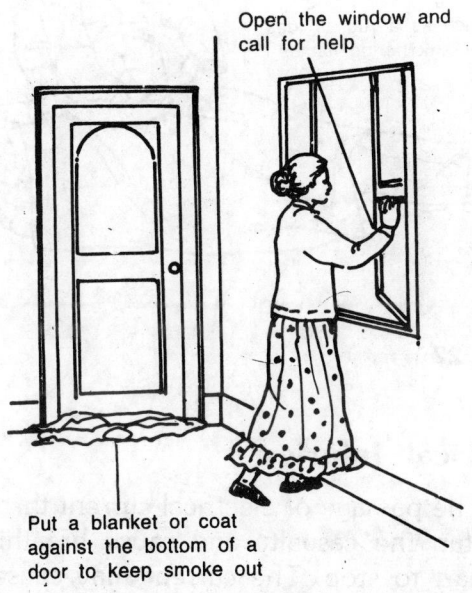

Open the window and call for help

Put a blanket or coat against the bottom of a door to keep smoke out

Figure 21

65

Clothing on fire

The casualty must be prevented from panicking and rushing outside. any movement or breeze will fan the flames.

1. Quickly lay the casualty down with the burning side uppermost and put off the flames by dousing the victim with water, or other non-inflammable liquid.

2. Wrap the casualty tightly in a coat, curtain blanket, rug or other heavy fabric. Then lay him on the ground. This starves the flames of oxygen (air) and puts them out.

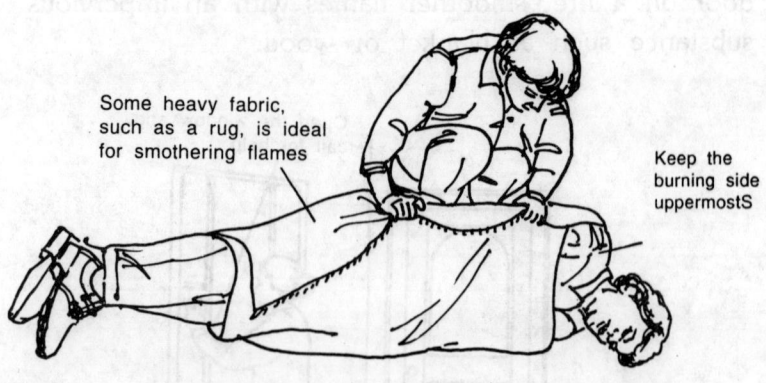

Some heavy fabric, such as a rug, is ideal for smothering flames

Keep the burning side uppermostS

Figure 22

Electrical Injuries

The passage of electrical current through the body may stun the casualty and cause breathing and even the heart to stop. The current may cause bruns, both where it enters the body and where it leaves the body to "earth".

Low voltage current

Domestic current as used in homes, offices, workshops, and shops, can cause serious injury, and even death. Many injuries result from faulty switches, frayed flex, or defects within an appliance itself. Young children are especially at risk.

You must be aware of the hazards of water, which is a dangerously good conductor of electricity. Handling an otherwise safe appliance with wet hands, or when standing on a wet floor, substantially increases the risk of a shock.

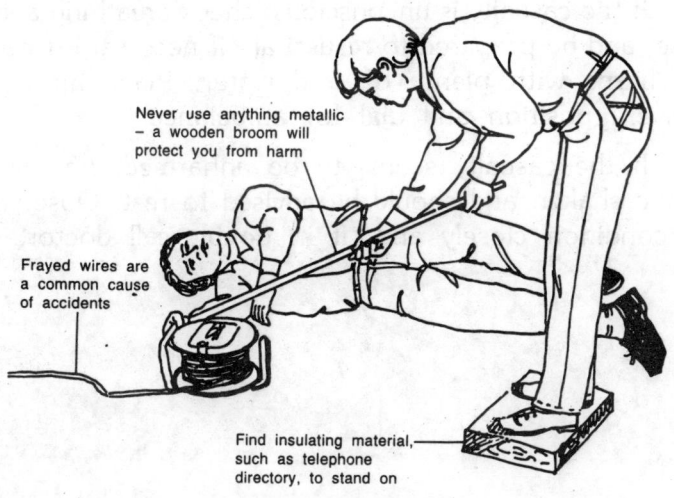

Never use anything metallic
– a wooden broom will
protect you from harm

Frayed wires are
a common cause
of accidents

Find insulating material,
such as telephone
directory, to stand on

Figure 23

First aid measures

1.   Break the contact by switching off the current, at the mains or meter if it can be reached easily. Otherwise, remove the plug, or wrench the cable free.

2. If you are unable to reach the cable, socket, or mains:

   a) Stand on dry insulating material such as a wooden box, a rubber or plastic mat, or thick pile of newspapers. Use a broom, wooden chair or stool to push the casualty's limbs away from the source.

   b) Without touching the casualty, loop rope around his feet or under the arms and pull him away from the source.

   c) As a last resort only, tug at the casualty's loose, dry clothing.

Once the current is broken:

If the casualty is unconscious, check breathing and pulse, and be prepared to resuscitate if necessary. Cool any burns with plenty of cold water. Place him in recovery position and dial for ambulance.

If the casualty seems to be unharmed, he may still be shaken and should be advised to rest. Observe his condition closely and, if in doubt, call doctor.

CARDIAC EMERGENCY

First Aid for Cardiopulmonary arrest

Establish unresponsiveness

1. When you first discover the victim, look at him closely. Shake him gently by the shoulders and shout "Are you okay?". This "shaking and shouting" will establish whether or not he is unconscious.

2. Observe A.B.C. of resuscitation - A = Airway, B = Breathing, C = Circulation.

Open the airway

1. Open the victim's airway. The most common cause of airway obstruction in an unconscious person is the tongue, which has relaxed and fallen into the airway

   a) Because the tongue is attached to the lower jaw, moving the lower jaw forward will lift the tongue away from the back of the throat, opening the airway

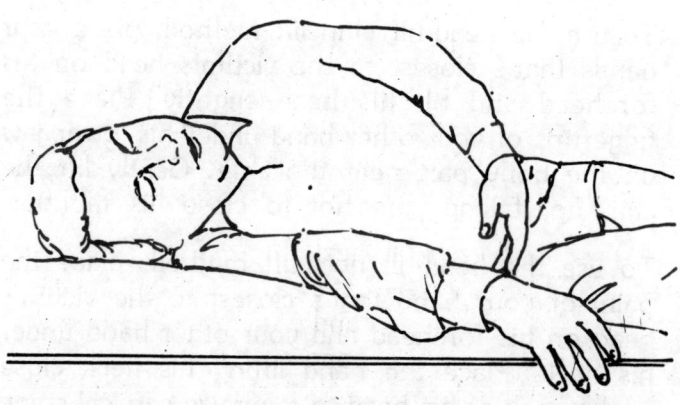

Figure 24 : First aid for cardiopulmonary arrest

69

b) You can use three methods to open the airway: the preferred head-tilt/chin-lift, the head-tilt/ neck-lift, or the jaw thrust without head-tilt.

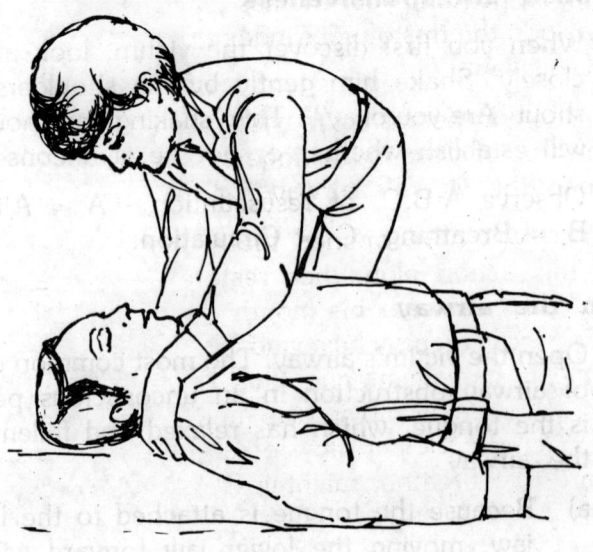

Figure 25

2. To use the head-tilt/chin lift method, place your hands that's closest to the victim's head on his forehead and tilt his head slightly. Place the fingertips of your other hand under his lower jaw on the bony part near the chin. Gently lift the chin up, taking care not to close his mouth.

3. To use the head-tilt/neck-lift method, place the palm of your hand that's closest to the victim's head on his forehead and your other hand under his neck. Place the hand lifting his neck close to the back of his head to minimize cervical-spine extension. Then gently press back on his forehead while lifting up and supporting his neck.

4. Use the jaw-thrust without head-tilt method if you suspect the victim has a neck or spine injury. Kneel at the victim's head, facing his feet. Place your thumbs on his mandible near the corners of his mouth, pointing your thumbs toward his feet. Then position the tips of your index fingers at the angles of his jaw.

Push your thumbs down while you lift upward with the tips of your index fingers. This action should open the victim's airway.

5. Once you have opened the victim's airway, see if this action alone has restored his breathing. Put your ear over his mouth and nose while you look forward his chest and abdomen. Listen for any air movement and look to see if his chest or abdomen is moving up and down. Feel with your cheek for any flow of air. If the victim has started to breathe, maintain his airway until help arrives.

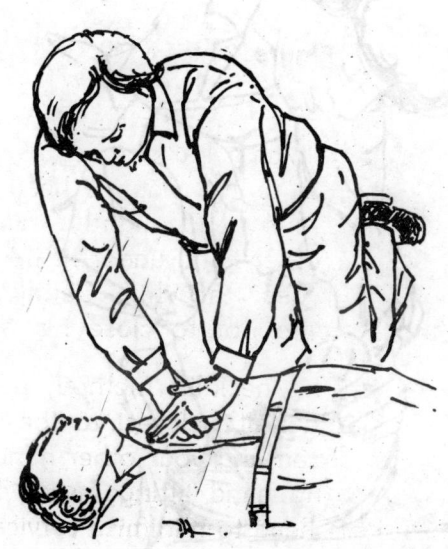

Figure 26

71

Restore breathing

1. If the victim hasn't started to breathe, close his nostrils with the thumb and index finger of your hand on his forehead.

2. Open your mouth wide and place it over the victim's mouth, sealing it tightly so no air can escape.

3. When you use the jaw-thrust method to open the airway, you must tuck your cheek under his nostrils.

4. Deliver four quick stairstep breaths

   a) Don't allow the victim to exhale between these breaths

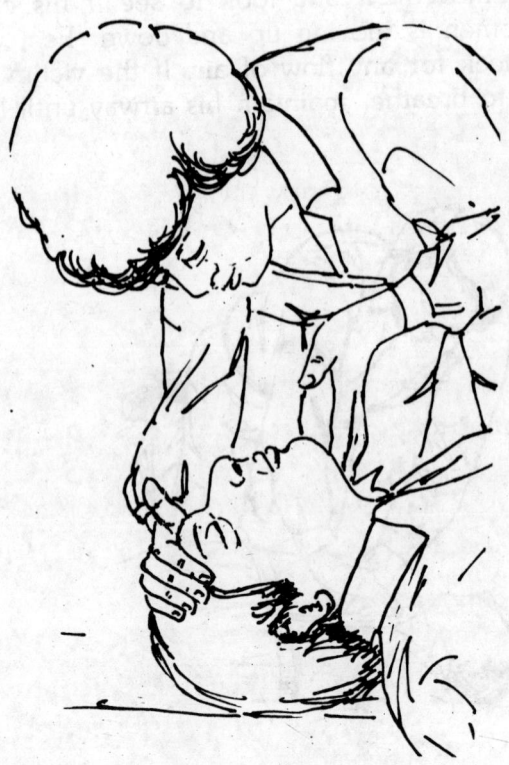

Figure 27

b) These four breaths maintain positive pressure in the airway. Even if the victim has stopped breathing for only for a short time, some of his lungs' alveoli may have collapsed. Positive pressure helps reinflate them.

When you see the victim's chest rise, then fall (after your fourth breath), you will know that air is entering and escaping his lungs.

If the victim wears dentures, keeping them in place will usually make ventilation easier. But if they are slipping, remove them.

Restore circulation

1. Now locate the victim's carotid pulse. To do so, keep your hand on his forehead to maintain the head-tilt position. Use your other hand to find the carotid artery on the side closest to you, in the groove beside the larynx. Use your index and middle fingers to gently palpate the artery for 5 to 10 seconds.

   If you find a pulse, don't give cardiac compressions but do ventilate the patient at a rate of one breath every seconds (12 breaths a minute). Continue to check his pulse after every 12 breaths.

   If you find no pulse, prepare to begin cardiac compression. Position yourself close to the victim's side, with your knees apart. This position gives you a broad base of support.

2. Use the fingers of your hand that's closest to the victim's feet to lower margin of his rib cage and trace the margin to the notch where the ribs meet the sternum.

3. Next, place your middle finger on the notch.

73

4. Place your index finger of the same hand next to your middle finger. Then place the heel of your other hand next to your index finger on the long axis of the sternum, as shown. This is the correct position for cardiac compression. If your hands are placed incorrectly, you may lacerate the victim's liver or fracture a rib.

5. Place the hand you used to locate the notch over the heel of your other hand. Interlock or extend your fingers to keep them off the victim's ribs and to maintain vertical pressure through the heel of the hand touching the sternum. Align your shoulders over your hands, keeping your elbows straight. Keeping your fingers off the ribs and your shoulders aligned ensures that you will compress downward, not laterally. Lateral compressions won't deliver sufficient pressure.

   Using the weight of your upper body, compress downward about 1.1/2 to 2 inches (3 to 5 cm), concentrating the pressure through the heels of your hands. Don't deliver bouncing compressions because they are less effective and could injure the victim. Then relax the pressure completely to let the victim's heart fill with blood. Don't remove your hands from his chest when you relax, or you will lose your hand position.

6. If you are the only rescuer, time your compressions at a rate of 80 a minute. Count, "One and two and three and four and five and ..." upto the count of fifteen. Then deliver two quick breaths without allowing the victim to exhale between them. (Actually, you will be delivering 60 compressions a minute, with the delay to ventilate the victim). Perform CPR for 1 minute, check the victim's pulse, then quickly telephone for help if none has arrived. Return quickly and resume CPR. If there is no phone available, continue CPR.

7. If a second rescuer arrives, ask her to call or go for help if you have not been able to do so. Then she can help you resuscitate the victim. (Of course, she must be trained in CPR if she is going to assist you).

8. Have the second rescuer get on the opposite side of the victim's airway, across from you. As she opens the victim's airway and tries to locate the carotid pulse, you continue giving compressions. If your compressions are strong enough, she should feel a pulse.

    When the second rescuer signals that she has found the pulse you are generating, stop your compressions for 5 seconds so she can see if the victim's heart is beating on its own.

9. If she can't discern a spontaneous pulse, she should deliver one breath. You can then resume compressions (approximately 60 a minute), while the second rescuer delivers a full breath on the upstroke of every fifth compressions. To assure that you work as a team, count out loud: "One, one thousand, two, one thousand, three, one thousand, four, one thousand, five, one thousand... " and so on. Have the second rescuer check for the victim's pulse every few minutes.

10. When you feel tired, tell the second rescuer you want to switch positions. To alert her, say: "Switch, one thousand, two, one thousand, five, one thousand". When you finish this count, the second rescuer should be delivering a full breath as you a move toward the victim's head.

11. When you get to his head, open his airway and assess his carotid pulse for 5 seconds. The second rescuer should get into position for cardiac compression.

12. If you can't feel a pulse, deliver one breath and tell the second rescuer to start the compressions. If you do find a pulse but the victim is not breathing, tell the second rescuer not to give any compressions. Continue giving the victim mouth-mouth ventilation and check his pulse every few minutes, in case his heart stops again.

Cardiopulmonary resuscitation for small children and infants is similar to that for adults. Generally, a child younger than a year is considered an infant, and one between 1 and 8 years old is considered a small child. Use adult CPR techniques for children older than 8 years.

In an emergency, of course, you are not going to delay CPR until you determine the child's age. Instead, consider his body size relation to the size of your hand. For example, if he looks too small to use both hands for cardiac compression, use the heel of one hand. If he is too small for that, use two or three fingers.

CPR for small children

1. Use the head-tilt/neck-lift (as shown) or head-tilt/chin-lift method to open the airway. You may need to use two or three fingers instead of your whole hand to lift the child's neck if it is very small.

2. If you use the head-tilt/chin-lift method, be careful not to close the child's mouth when you lift his chin. Also, be sure your fingers are not pressing on the soft tissue under his chin, which may cause oedema and subsequent airway obstruction.

3. If the child's face is large enough, maintain a tight seal by pinching his nostrils (as shown) and placing your mouth over his. If he has a small face, place your mouth over his mouth and nose. When ventilating, give only enough air to make the child's chest rise.

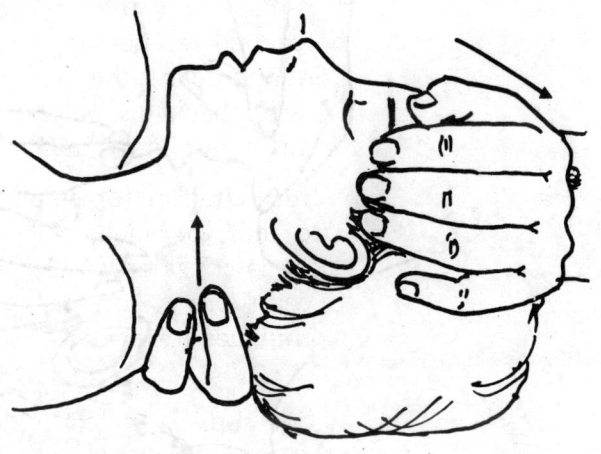

Figure 28

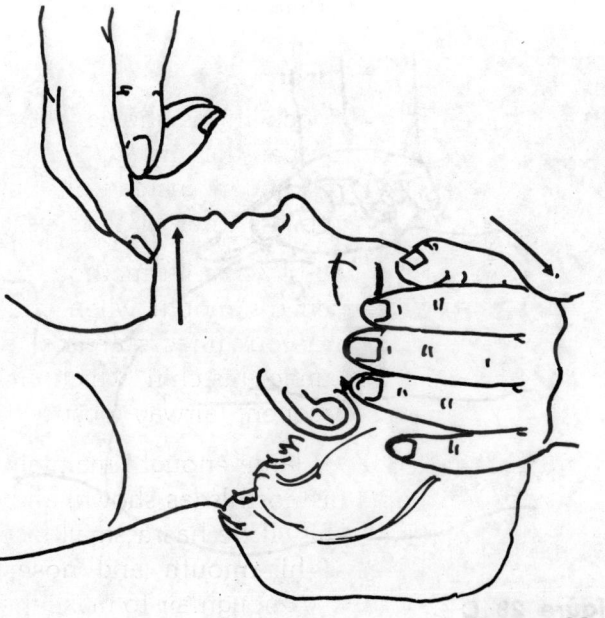

Figure 28 A

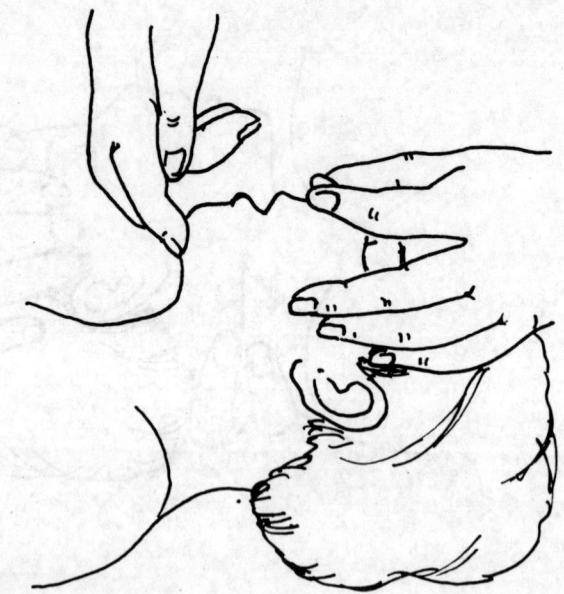

Figure 28 B

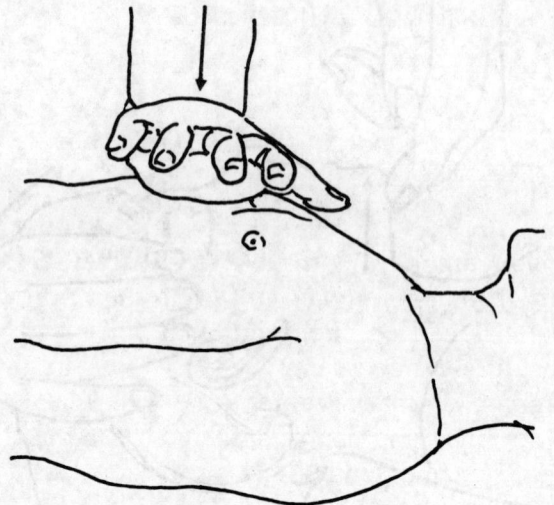

Figure 28 C

78

4. Try to palpate the child's carotid pulse. If you find a pulse, do not give cardiac compression but do ventilate the child at a rate of one breath every 4 seconds. If you can't locate a pulse, find the proper location for compression. Use the same technique you would for an adult. Then compress about 1 to 1.½ inches (2.5 to 3.8 cm), using the heel of one hand (as shown).

Give 80 compressions a minute, with a breath after every fifth compression. Your count should be: "One and two and three and four and five and one..." and so on. This rate and ratio are the same if you have a second rescuer helping you, but the second rescuer should ventilate on the upstroke of the fifth compression.

CPR for infants

1. When you tilt an infant's head, you will lift up his back as well. So before opening an infant's airway, place a rolled towel of your hand closest to his feet beneath his back to support it. Then gently tilt his head back. You don't need to lift his neck.

2. Cover both his mouth and nose with your mouth. To ventilate, give only small breaths - just enough to make his chest rise.

3. If you are having trouble ventilating the infant, his stomach may be distended, limiting chest expansion. Don't relieve gastric distension unless absolutely necessary, because the infant may aspirate stomach contents. But if his abdomen is so tense you can't ventilate, turn him onto his right side and gently press on his epigastric region.

Gastric distension is caused by delivering too much air, so give only enough air to make the infant's chest rise.

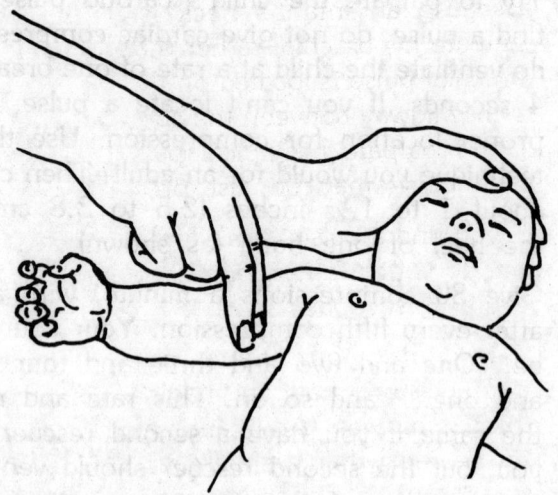

Figure 29

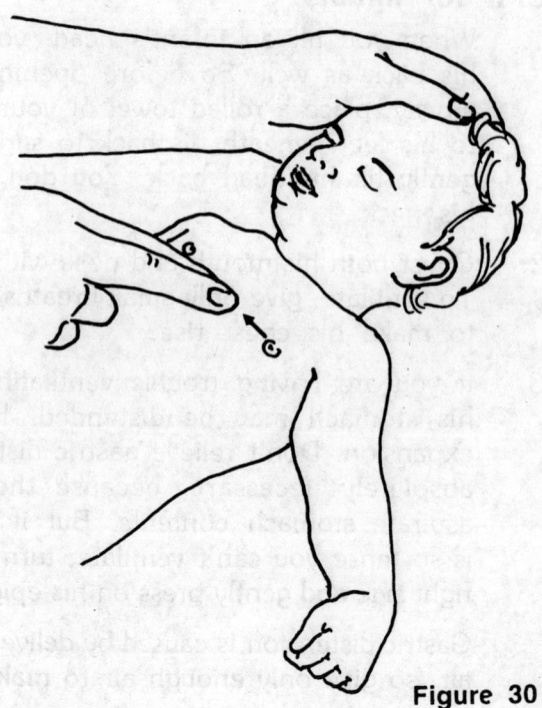

Figure 30

4. Because an infant's neck is short and chubby, palpate his brachial rather than carotid pulse. The brachial pulse is located on the inside of the upper arm, midway between the shoulder and the elbow. Don't palpate his apical pulse - what you think is a pulse may be just precordial activity.

   If you find a pulse, don't give cardiac compression but do ventilate the infant at a rate of one breath every 3 seconds.

5. To locate your hand position for cardiac compression, draw an imaginary line between the infant's nipples. (An infant's heart is located higher in the chest than a small child's or adult's). Place two or three fingers in the middle of this line. Deliver about 100 compressions a minute, giving a breath after every five compressions. Count to yourself: "One, two, three, four, five" (even though you are alone). Because an infant is so small, one rescuer along can try to resuscitate him.

POISONING

Some substances when taken into the body in fairly large quantities, can be dangerous to health or can cause death. Such substances are called poisons. They may be taken with a view to committing suicide or may be given to persons by enemies deliberately or taken by mistake.

Swallowed poisons

Sometimes acids, alkalies, disinfectants etc., are swallowed by mistake. They burn the lips, tongue, throat, food passage and stomach and cause great pain. Other swallowed poisons cause vomiting, pain and later on diarrhoea. Poisonous fungi-berries, metallic poisons and stale food belong to the latter group. Some swallowed poisons affect the nervous system. To this ʒroup belong:

a) Alcoholic drink when taken in large quantities.

b) Tablets for sleeping, tranquilizers and pain killing drugs. All these victims must be considered as seriously ill. The symptoms are either fits or coma. Some poison act on nervous system.

Inhaled poisons

Fumes or gases from charcoal stoves, household gas, motor exhausts and smoke from explosions etc., cause choking which may result in unconsciousness in addition to difficult in breathing.

Injected poisons

Poisons get into the body through injection, bites of poisonous snakes and rabies dogs or stings by scorpions and insects. Danger to life is again by choking and coma.

First aid in poisoning

1. Poisoning is a serious matter. Patient must be removed to a hospital or a doctor be sent for at once with a note of the findings and if possible, the name of the person.

2. Preserve packets or bottles which you suspect contained the poison and also any vomits, sputum etc., for the doctor to deal with.

3. If unconscious

   a) Do not induce vomiting

   b) Make the casualty lie on his back on a hard, flat bed without any pillow and turn the head to one side. As there is no pressure on the stomach and the gullet is horizontal, the vomited matter will not get into the voice box and the tongue will not close the air passage. This is also the best positive for giving artificial respiration, if needed.

   c) Sometimes when there is excess of vomiting, the three quarters prone posture will make things easier for the casualty.

   d) If breathing is very slow or stopped, start artificial respiration and keep it up, till the doctor comes.

4. If conscious,

   a) Aid vomiting by tickling the back of throat or make him drink tepid water mixed with 2 tablespoons of common salt for a tumble, of water.

   b) Even if conscious, when the poison is a corrosive, do not induce vomiting.

Signs of corrosive poisoning

Lips, mouth and skin show gray white or yellow patches which are to be looked for acids, alkalies etc., cause such burns.

Management

Factories which use certain poisons shall have the respective antidotes ready and displayed in an easily available place. The personnel should be taught about the use of antidotes - so that, anyone can render assistance in case of emergency.

5. The poison must be diluted by giving large quantities of cold water. This will dilute the irritant and delay absorption and will replace fluid lost by vomiting. Tender coconut water will be even better, as this will be a food and also a diuretic.

6. Soothing drinks should be given. Milk, egg beaten and mixed with water or sojee congee are good for the purpose.

BITES AND STINGS

Snake bite

There are more than 2,500 different kinds of snakes. Only about 200 of them are venomous. All snake bites are not fatal. Only a very small quantity of the venom might have been injected. Most people will not die because of the venom but from fear.

Figure 31

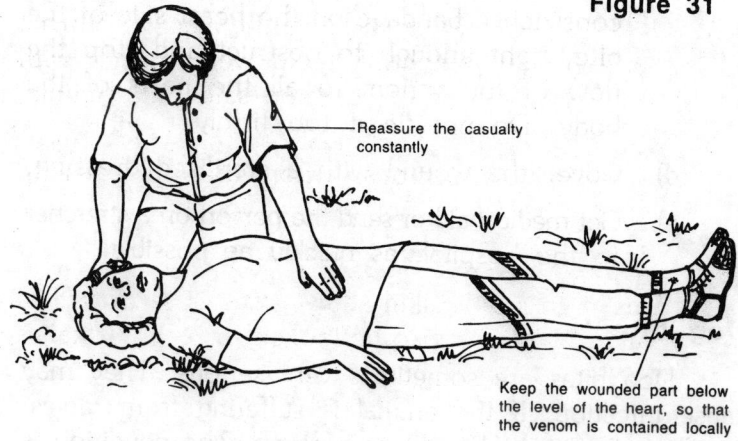

Reassure the casualty constantly

Keep the wounded part below the level of the heart, so that the venom is contained locally

Aim of first-aid

a) To reassure the person

b) To stop spreading of the venom

c) To obtain medical aid.

Figure 32

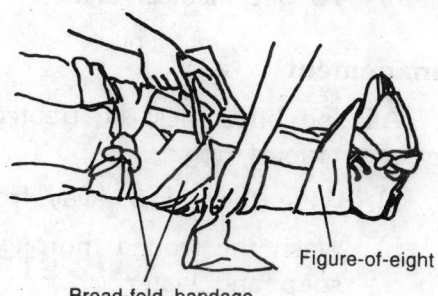

Figure-of-eight

Broad-fold bandage

Management

a) Lay the patient down, give him complete rest, calm and reassure him, never make him walk.

b) Wash the wound with soap and water, flush the wound with a lot of water.

85

c) If the bite is on the arm or leg, apply a constrictive bandage on the heart side of the bite, tight enough to obstruct and stop the flow of the venom to all the parts of the body. Do not tie it too firmly.

d) Cover the wound with a sterilized dressing.

e) Get medical aid or send the person on a stretcher to the hospital, as quickly as possible.

Dog bite

Dog bites are sometimes very serious. They may cause infection. If the animal is suffering from rabies, it will be transmitted to these persons. The condition is known as Hydrophobia. Therefore, the dog should not be killed. It must be chained and kept under observation for ten days. If the dog is healthy after this period, there is no danger of rabies.

Aim of first-aid

a) To prevent rabies or other infections.

b) To get medical aid.

Management

All dog bites must be treated as potentially as bite by a rabies dog.

a) Wipe the saliva away from the wound.

b) Wash the wound thoroughly, with plenty of soap and water.

c) Cover the wound with a dry, sterile dressing. Do not put carbolic acid, nitric acid etc., on the wound within 1/2 hours of bite.

d) Get medical aid or send the patient to the hospital for proper treatment of the wound and also the casualty.

Insect bite and stings

Stings of mites, ticks and leeches:

Mites, ticks and leeches are found in marshes and jungles. They attach themselves firmly to the skin. Mites and ticks may carry Typhus and may transmit it to the person. Leeches are normally harmless, but they suck blood from the victim.

Management

1. Don't try to remove the insects manually, their mouth parts may remain in the skin and may cause inflammation and infection.

2. Put the burning end of a cigarette to the body of the ticks and leeches, they will fall off.

3. Application of salt results in leech dropping off.

4. Mites are so small that they cannot be easily seen to be removed.

5. Clean the area with methylated spirit.

6. Apply weak ammonia or bicarbonate of soda or antihistamine content. This will relieve irritation.

Stings of bees, rasps, fleas and hornets

The stings of bees, rasps etc., can cause a lot of pain. The area may swell. Sometimes, the person may suffer from shock.

Management

a) A sting should be removed with forceps or with the tip of a sterilized needle.

b) Apply weak ammonia or bicarbonate of soda or antihistamine ointment to the area. This will relieve the pain.

Household poisons

Many substances found in and about the home, can be poisonous. These include liquid soap, some cosmetics, white spirit, rat poison etc. Children who are not aware of the consequences of eating these substances, become an easy prey to these poisons. The symptoms and signs vary according to the nature of these poisons. In most cases, vomiting and abdominal pain are common symptoms. Children take medicines, found in medicine cabinets without knowing the consequences. Even though, most of them are not poisonous, if taken as per the directions of the doctor. If taken in larger doses than suggested, they act as poisons. So, always make sure that all bottles and jars containing poisonous substances are kept out of reach of children.

In recent years, the pattern of poisoning has changed and today, the overall incidence is roughly,

1. Barbiturates 40%, (Sleeping tablets)

2. Aspirin 20%,

3. The rest 20%.

It is important to distinguish between those poisons which are corrosive and burn the mouth and those which are not.

While giving first aid the first thing to do is to ensure that respiration and circulation are maintained. Then, it is necessary to decide as to what type of poison has been used. If a corrosive which will cause burning of lips, mouth and tongue or if paraffin or petroleum product which, though harmless in the stomach, would cause grave damage if inhaled. Send quickly to the hospital. With all other poisons, the patient should be made to vomit by giving two table spoonfuls of salt in a glass of warm water or two teaspoonfuls of mustard in a glass of warm water. Send the patient to the hospital as quickly as possible.

Specific Poisons

Barbiturates

This is usually suicidal, though it may be accidental in children. They may eat sleeping tablets carelessly left around by the parents. The patient goes in to a deep sleep and then into coma with respiratory depression, low blood pressure, a quick and feeble pulse and a cold clammy skin. Emetic, given soon after the tablets are taken, will be effective as the drug has sedative action on the stomach. Early admission to the hospital should be arranged. In the meanwhile, the first aider must be on the look out for respiratory failure and be prepared to give artificial respiration.

Aspirin

It is used in large doses as a suicidal attempt. Its repeated and prolonged usage for the treatment of pain may irritate the lining of the stomach and produce haemorrhage. If taken in large doses, it may produce vomiting and its effect on the central nervous system is to produce confusion, convulsions, sweating, over breathing etc. Extensive gastric bleeding may also occur. The emetic is effective because of the slow rate of absorption. So, a doctor may wash out the stomach with good results.

Carbon monoxide

Common sources are domestic gas, exhaust fumes from petrol engines etc. It may be accidental or suicidal. Giddiness, headache and tightness of the chest, loss of use of lower limbs and unconsciousness are common symptoms. The patient will have a characteristic pink appearance and may have stopped breathing.

Poisonous plants

Certain plants grown in our garden, as well as, in the forest are dangerous if eaten or comes into contact with them. Laburnum, deadly night shade and death cap fungus are more common examples of plants which can poison the system. The severity of the condition will depend on how much is consumed.

If it is found that the patient has consumed poisonous plant, you must maintain an open air way and remove the patient to the hospital.

Food poisoning

This is due to the contamination of food by bacteria. It may also be due to incorrect cooking and storing. The most common bacteria present is staphylococci. This multiplies in food and produce a poisonous substance which cause dysentery like illness. Symptoms of food poisoning depend upon the type of poisoning. The patient feels nauseated and may already be vomiting. The patient may be suffering from abdominal pain and may have headache. At a later stage, diarrhoea may develop. There may appear symptoms of shock. Seek immediate medical aid. Follow the general treatment for poisoning. Make sure, the patient rests. Give him plenty of fluids to drink. If you have any doubt, arrange removal to hospital.

Drug poisoning

This is caused by an accidental over dose of drug abuse. Drug abuse may be defined as the self administration of a drug in a manner that is not according to approved medical or social patterns. Drugs can be inhaled, swallowed or injected into the body. Drugs commonly abused; narcotics, depressants, stimulants and hallucinogens.

The symptoms depend on the drug and the quantity taken. The pupils of the eye may be abnormally dilated or contracted.

Narcotics are injected or taken in tablet form or inhaled. Breathing becomes difficult and, eventually, stop. The patient may have injection marks on the front of one or both the arms. When depressants are taken, breathing will be shallow. Patient's skin feel cold and clammy. Pulse will be weak and rapid. The patient may be unconscious. When stimulants are taken, the patient will be excitable and sweating profusely. The patient may be suffering from tremors and hallucinations. If the patient has taken hallucinogens, he will be anxious and sweating. The patient may be behaving strangely. When an over dose of aspirin has been taken, the patient has abdominal pain and may be vomiting. He may be depressed and drowsy. He may complain of ringing in the ears. There will be difficulty in breathing. He may be sweating profusely. His pulse will be full.

While treating such patients, follow the general treatment for poisoning. Arrange for urgent removal to the hospital. You must be prepared to resuscitate.

Alcohol poisoning

Alcohol depresses the central nervous system. It affects different people in different ways. The drug affects the areas of higher reasoning within the brain. As the concentration of alcohol in blood increases, the behaviour of the patient becomes exaggerated and coordination will be affected.

Patient's breath may smell of alcohol. Patient may be vomiting. The patient may be partly conscious or fully unconscious. The patient may be breathing deeply. Face will be moist and flushed. Pulse will be full and bounding. In later stages of unconsciousness, pulse may become rapid but weak. Breathing will be shallow. The patient's face appears dry and look bloated. Eyes will be blood shot and pupils may be dilated.

Maintain a open air way. If the patient becomes unconscious or vomiting is likely. Place her in the recovery position. If necessary, complete resuscitation. If there is any doubt about the condition of the patient make arrangements to remove the patient to the hospital.

Industrial poisons

As a result of failure of a chemical plant, the workers may come in contact with dangerous chemicals or gases. Most common industrial poisons are gases. There are so many different poisonous substances that, it is impossible to give a list. Always remember that any patient suffering from the effects of gas or toxic fumes, needs air. While giving first aid, be sure that you yourself are not trapped in any fumes that remain in the area. Do not try to rescue a patient trapped in an enclosed space, if you are not equipped with and practiced in the use of breathing apparatus and life lines.

Some common poisons and their first aid

1. **Acetyl salicylic acid :** Found in Aspirin, APC tabs - vomiting to be induced. Give 1 teaspoon of soda bicarb in one glass of water.

2. **Concentrated acid :** Found in hospitals, laboratories etc. - Vomiting should not be induced. Excess of water to be given to weaken the acid. One table spoon of milk of magnesia may be given in one glass of water. Chalk and soda bicarb may also be used.

3. **Concentrated alkali :** Found in hospital, laboratory and some factories - No vomiting to be induced, give excess of water to weaken the alkali. One table spoonful of vinegar, orange and lemon.

4. **Arsenic:** It is found in rat killing medicine and insecticides - Vomiting should be induced. Sweet beverages, like milk, egg white or solution of wheat flour in water may be given.

92

5. **Atropine or Belladonna ointment :** Eye ointment, eyedrops - Vomiting to be induced. Tea or coffee may be given to drink.

6. **Carbon monoxide :** Found in gas burner smoke, smokes of motors - Artificial respiration may be given. Oxygen may be given, if available.

7. **Hypnotics :** Hypnotics and tabs and powder to get relief from pain - A tablespoon of epsom salt in a glass of water. Hot tea or coffee may be given. The person should be kept awake. Artificial respiration may be given.

8. **Disinfectants :** No vomiting. Epsom (cresol, lysol, dettol etc.) Salt may be given in one glass of water or paraffin.

9. **Lead :** Found in some colours and hair dyes. Vomiting should be induced. One spoon of epsom salt in a glass of water may be given.

10. **Mercury :** Milk may be given after giving egg white mixed with water. Then induce vomiting.

11. **Morphine :** Found in hospitals, house and agricultural fields. Vomiting to be induced. Some grains of potassium permanganate may be given in one glass of water to drink. Hot tea or coffee may be given to drink. The person should be kept awake. He may be kept covered.

12. **Paraffin and petrol (kerosene) :** Found in house, garages and factories - Induce vomiting immediately. Excess amount of water may be given to drink. If the person has taken kerosene, liquid paraffin in one glass of water may be given.

13. **Phosphorus :** Found in rat killing medicine - Vomiting may be induced and some grains of potassium permanganate in a glass of water to drink.

14. **Prussic acid** : Found in photography and electroplating and bitter almond oil - Immediately vomiting should be induced, artificial respiration may be resorted to.

15. **Strychnine** : Found in some insecticides - Induce vomiting before the cramps are started. Let the patient be peaceful. His severe movements should not be controlled by hand. Artificial respiration, if respiration has stopped.

Antidotes

Charcoal can be given in water down a stomach or nasogastric tube as an absorbent and is effective in reducing the absorption of tricyclic anti depressants and paracetamol. Whole blood filtration is recommended for paraquat poisoning. It must be done, as soon as the poison is identified in urine.

Fullers earth and bentonite are other absorbent media which have been recommended for paraquat. 150g. in milk, water or squash may be given at first contact without fear of harm and with possible benefit. A new gleam of hope is available from cardiff for treatment of paraquat poisoning. In radiation of affected lungs with low doses of τ rays labeled with cobalt-60. Mannitol 20% is currently recommended for fuller earth. 250 ml should be given by nasogastric tube followed by magnesium sulphate by mouth to increase excretion of absorbed paraquat.

Points to remember

A poison is any substance that, if taken into the body, can cause temporary or permanent damage. Poison enters the body through the mouth by eating or drinking poisonous substances. It may enter through lungs by inhaling household or industrial gases. It may enter the body by injection into the skin as a result of bites and stings. It is always best to shift the patient to the nearest hospital, as quickly as possible.

LOSS OF CONSCIOUSNESS

Any interference with the normal functioning of the brain and the nerves brings about loss of sensitivity. An unconscious state indicates not only that there might be some disease or injury of the brain but serious injuries and diseases elsewhere in the body.

Unconsciousness due to injuries are of two kinds

a) Partial when it is called stupor and

b) Complete when it is known as coma.

Tests for degree of unconscious state

a) When spoken to the casualty, may not respond while in stupor, he can be roused with difficult, in coma there is no responses at all.

b) In stupor, one cannot open the eye lids as the casualty will resist this attempt. But in coma, lids can be opened without any resistances.

c) Pupil test:

Pupil is the round opening in the centre of the Iris. In stupor, caused by diseases or injuries, the pupil

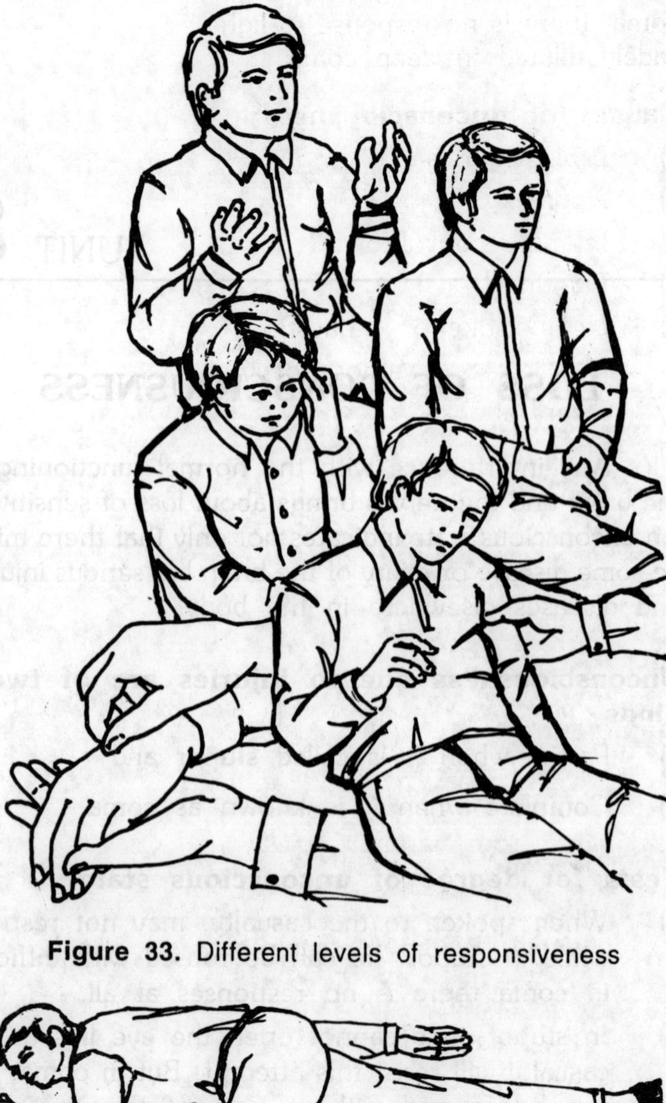

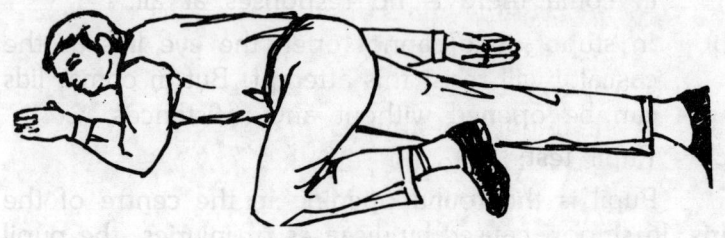

Figure 33. Different levels of responsiveness

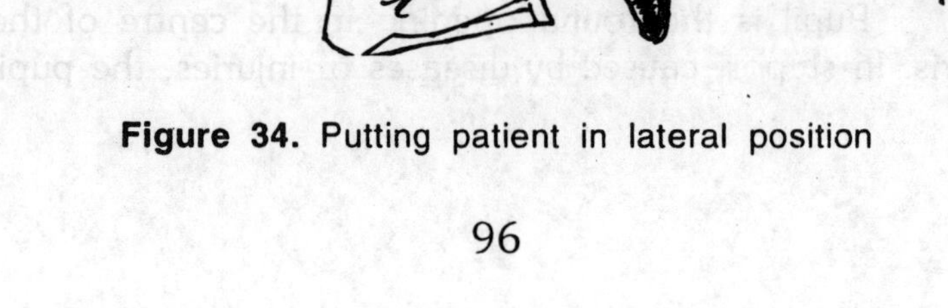

Figure 34. Putting patient in lateral position

contract when light is made to fall on it. But in coma, there is no response to light. In fact, it is often widely dilated in deep coma.

Causes of unconsciousness

a) Brain injuries
b) Apoplexy
c) Infantile convulsions.
d) Fainting.
e) Heat stroke or exhaustion.
f) Diabetes or overdose of insulin.
g) Heart attacks.
h) Hysteria.
i) Epilepsy.
j) Shock
k) Haemorrhage.
l) Acute fever
m) Poisons.

Management

a) See that there is a free supply of fresh air and that the air passages are free. Take the casualty away from harmful gases, if any. If inside the room, open doors and windows. Remove false teeth. Above all, keep back crowds, they only obstruct. Watch for symptoms for shock.

b) Loosen tight clothing up at neck, chest and waist.

c) If the weather is cold, wrap blankets around the body.

d) If breathing has stopped or about to stop, turn the casualty into the required posture and start artificial respiration.

e) Breathing may be noisy or quiet. If not noisy, let the casualty lie on his back. Raise the shoulder

97

slightly by a pad, turn the head to one side, watch for sometime. If breathing becomes difficult or gets obstructed, change the posture to ease breathing. If breathing is noisy, turn casualty to three quats prone position and support in this position with pads.

f)   Apply specific treatment for the cause of unconsciousness.

g)   Watch continuously for any changes in the condition. Do not leave the casualty until he is passed on to medical hands.

h)   No form of drinks should be given in the conditions.

i)   It is best to remove the casualty to a sheltered place on a stretcher.

j)   On return to consciousness, wet the lips with water. If there is no thoracic or abdominal injury, sips of water also can be given.

Asphyxia

Asphyxia also otherwise called suffocation, is a condition in which the lungs do not get sufficient supply of air for breathing. If this continues for some minutes, breathing and heart action stop, and death occurs.

Causes of Asphyxia

This is a fatal condition which occurs, if there is not enough oxygen available for the tissues of the body. Such lack may be due to an insufficient amount of oxygen in the air breathed in or any interference with or injury to the respiratory system. There are many conditions which can result in Asphyxia. Some of them are,

1.   Obstructed air way due to the tongue falling into the back of the throat in an unconscious casualty, Food, vomit or other foreign matter present in the airway.

2. Fluid in the air passages.

3. Compression of the wind pipe by hanging or strangulation.

4. Compression of the chest.

5. Injury to lungs.

6. Injury to the chest walls.

7. Fits, preventing adequate breathing.

8. Laryngeal occlusion by food.

9. Head injuries.

10. Severe acute asthma

11. Drowning

12. Facial injuries

13. Anaphylaxis strings of wasp and bee

14. Angio neurotic oedema.

15. Epiglottitis (Croup)

General symptoms of asphyxia are,
1. Difficulty in breathing
2. Breathing may become noisy - snoring or gurgling
3. Frothing at the mouth
4. Blueness of face, lips and finger nails (cyanosis)
5. Confusion
6. Reduction in the level of responsiveness
7. Unconsciousness
8. Stoppage of breathing

General Treatment

Remove the cause of asphyxia and open the airway - Let him get enough fresh air. If the patient is unconscious, open his air way and check breathing. Check breathing rate, pulse rate and the level of responsiveness. Obtain medical aid as soon as possible.

Heat stroke

This is caused by every high environmental temperature or feverish illness like, malaria etc. It would raise the body temperature to a high degree and the body cannot control its temper by sweating etc. It can also be caused by prolonged confinement in a hot atmosphere. Heat stroke is due to a failure of the temperature regulating mechanism of the body. Its on set is sudden with changes in consciousness delirium, convulsions and coma. The body temperature rises above 40.6°C and no sweating. The onset may preceded by such warning signs as restlessness, aggressive behaviour and incoordinated actions. The skin is very hot and dry. The lips and face are congested. Pulse and breathing are both rapid.

Symptoms

The patient complains of headache, dizziness etc. The patient becomes restless. Unconsciousness may develop rapidly. The patient is hot with a temperature more than 40°C. Pulse is full and bounding. Breathing may be noisy.

The sole aim of first aid in such a situation is to reduce the patients temperature as quickly as possible and obtain medical aid.

We have to bring down his body temperature quickly. Keep the casualty in the coolest possible place. Remove clothing and sprinkle cool water on his body or wrap him in a thin wet sheet and fan him. The temperature begins to fall but it should not get lower than 102°F. After this stage is reached, wrap him in a dry sheet and fan him, so that, the temperature does not rise up again. On recovery, remove him to a cool

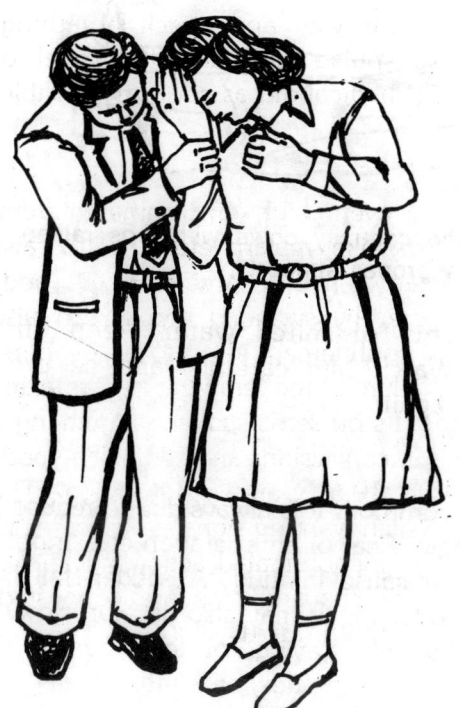

Figure 35.
Helping the
patient

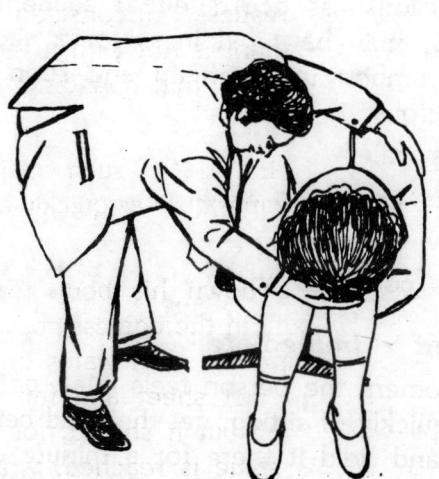

Figure 36. Allowing the patient to sit down

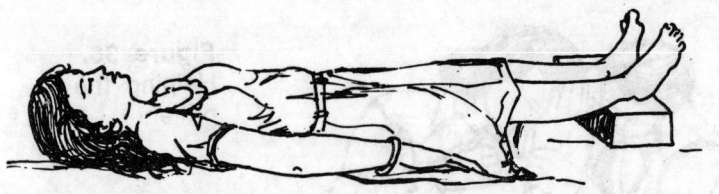

Figure 37. Laying the casualty down with legs raised on proper support

place, give him plenty of salted water, keep him comfortable warm. Watch him carefully and be prepared to treat him again.

Fainting

Fainting is very common. It is always due to reduced blood supply to the brain. Fear of an operation etc., fright, sad news, or pain can cause fainting. A sudden fall in blood pressure can produce it. It may also develop slowly in weak persons or people staying for long period in hot or stuffy places as in parades or stuffy rooms.

Signs and symptoms

a) Unconsciousness occurs either suddenly or the casualty, may have giddiness for a second, the body crumbles into a heap and soon becomes unconscious.

b) Face is pale.

c) Pulse is weak and slow.

d) Shallow breathing.

e) Skin is cold and sticky.

Management - Immediate

a) The moment the person feels faint, get his head down quickly. If sitting, get the head between the knees and hold it there for a minute or two. It may be necessary to lay him down, with the head at a slightly lower level than the feet.

b)   Hold smelling salt, if available, in front of the nose.

Later

c)   If seen later, the casualty will have become un-conscious, Lay him down as described above.

d)   See that there is plenty of fresh air, ask the on-lookers to disperse.

e)   Loosen clothing at waist, chest and neck.

f)   After recovery, only slowly raise the head then make him get up and sit down.

g)   Give sips of orange juice or tea or coffee or even water.

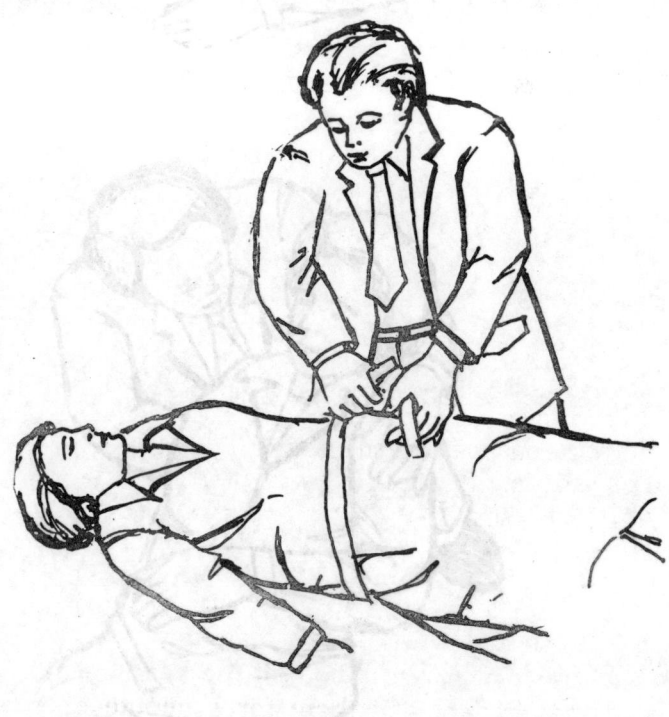

Figure 38. Loosening the clothes

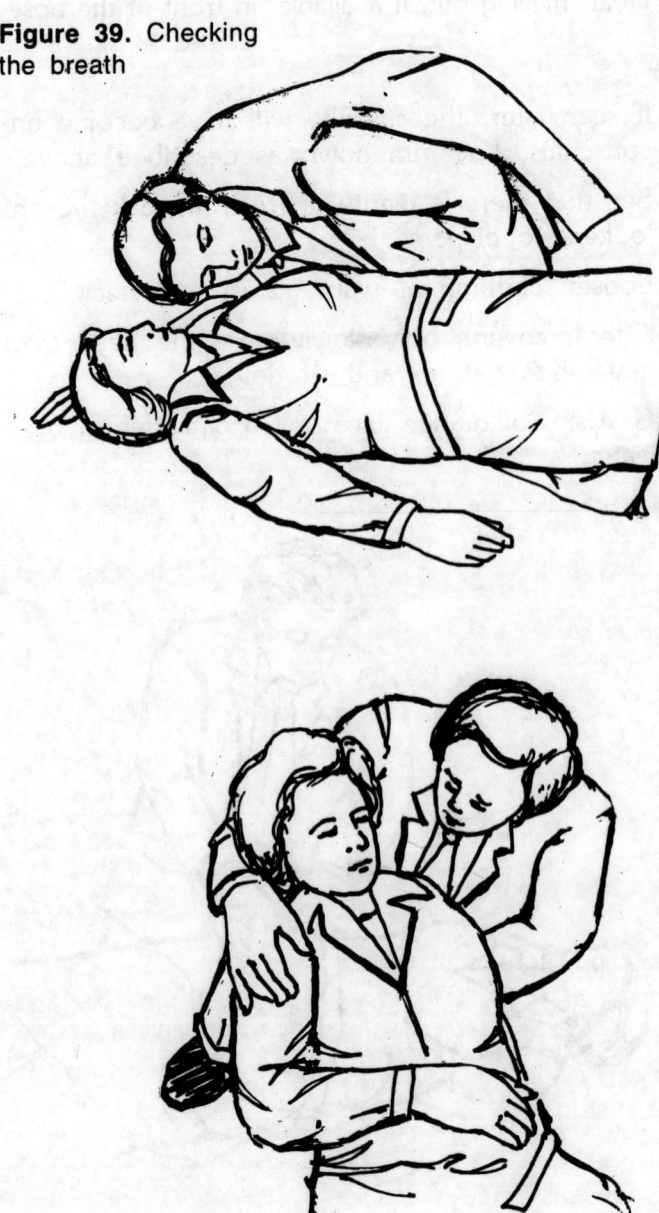

Figure 39. Checking the breath

Figure 40. Raising the patient gradually

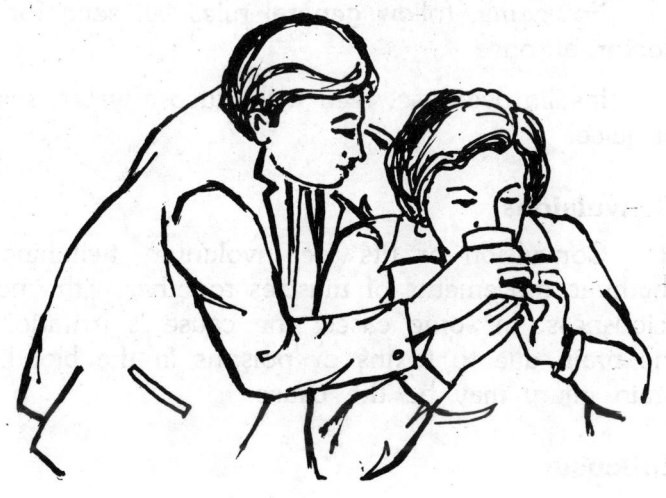

Figure 41. Giving liquid orally

Stupor

Is when the casualty can be roused with difficulty, or when the person is unconscious due to partial injuries.

Coma

Diabetic coma and over dose of insulin.

Signs and symptoms

The signs of diabetic coma is that the skin will be dry. The casualty will breathe deep and sighing. He may smell of acetone and he will be unconsciousness or stupor.

In overdose of insulin coma, the skin will be moist and the casualty may sweat. His breathing will be shallow and quiet. There will not be any smell of any sort, and the casualty may have fainted but very rarely he will become unconscious.

105

Management

For coma, follow general rules but send for the doctor at once.

Insulin overdose, feed with glucose water, sweets or juice.

Convulsions

Convulsion or fits are involuntary twitching or rhythmic movements of muscles together with unconsciousness. In some cases, the cause is irritation of the brain due to toxins or poisons in the blood, or brain injury may be the cause.

Epilepsy

This is a disease, usually, of young people. The cause may be injury to the brain at birth, or there may be a family tendency. Fits may occur at any time and in between, the person seems healthy.

In minor epilepsy, the casualty suddenly becomes unconscious for a few seconds, with eyes fixed and starting. He may then carry on with what he was doing, as though, nothing had happened.

A major epileptic fit may start with a headache, restlessness and a feeling that he is going to have a fit. The fit has four stages:

1. The person suddenly falls down unconscious, sometimes with a cry.

2. The eyes turn upwards, the breath is held, and the body becomes stiff for about half a minute.

3. Muscles twitch and then there are convulsive movements of the limbs, head and jaw. The tongue may be bitten. Breathing becomes heavy and there is frothing at the mouth and he may bite his tongue and urine may be passed.

106

4. Convulsions stop and the casualty is in a coma, or in stupor, he may act in a strange manner not knowing what he is doing.

   a) Protect the casualty from danger, such as, fire, sharp stones, water etc.

   b) Prevent the tongue from being bitten by placing a padded piece of wood, key, spoon or similar object between the back teeth on one side. These may be prepared during the rigid stage (stage 2).

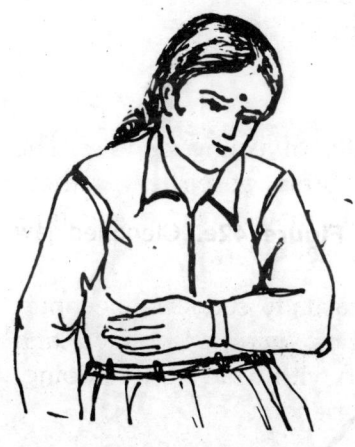

Figure 42a. Victim having an aura

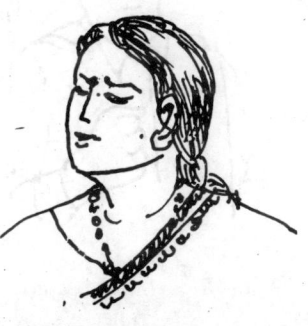

Figure 42b. Different stages of aura

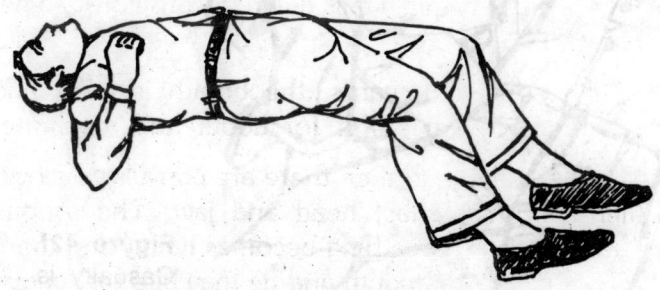

Figure 42c. Body becoming rigid

107

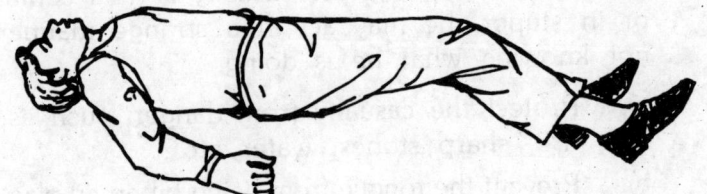

Figure 42d. Arched back

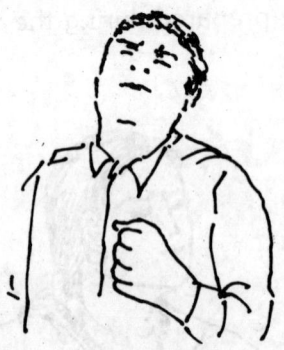

Figure 42e. Clenched jaw

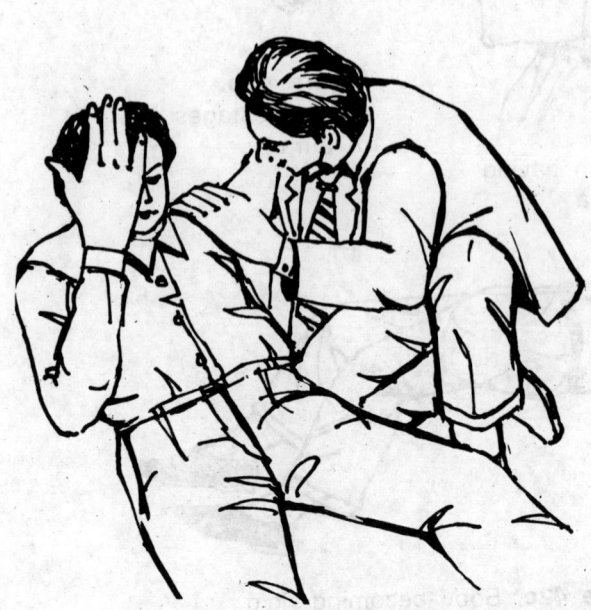

Figure 42f.
Casualty is
allowed to rest

5. Do not try to restrain movements, except to prevent injury.

6. Wipe froth from the mouth.

7. Follow the general rules for treatment of an unconscious person.

8. When he is recovered, give a warm sweet drink.

9. The person with epilepsy should see a doctor. If he has an order for tablets, he should take them regularly to avoid getting fits.

DROWNING

Drowning is the result of complete immerse of the nose and mouth in water. Water enters the windpipe and lungs, clogging the lungs completely. The aim is to get the casualty on to dry land with minimum danger to yourself.

Choose the safest way to rescue the casualty. If possible stay on land and reach with your hand a stick or a branch or throw a rope or float.

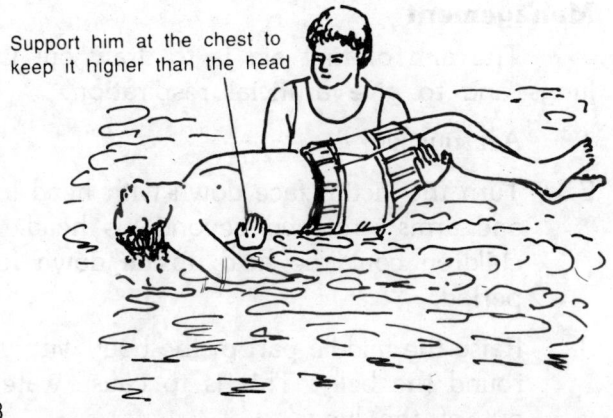

Support him at the chest to keep it higher than the head

Figure 43

Swim to the casualty and tow him only if you are a trained life-saver, or if the casualty is unconscious, it is safer to wade, if you can, than to swim.

When bringing the casualty out of water, carry him with his head lower than his chest, to minimise the dangers of vomiting.

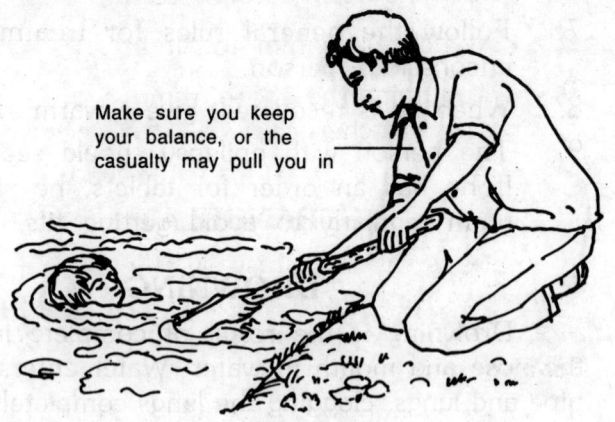

Make sure you keep your balance, or the casualty may pull you in

Figure 44

Treat for drowning and effects of cold.

Take or send the casualty to hospital even if he seems to have recovered well.

Management

The aim of first aid is to draw out water from lungs and to give artificial respiration.

1. Act quickly

2. Turn the victim face down with head to one side and arms stretched beyond his head. Infants or children could be held upside down for a short period.

3. Raise the middle part of the body with your hands round the belly. This is to cause water to draw out of the lungs.

4. Give artificial respiration until breathing comes back to normal. This may have to go on for as long as two hours.

5. Remove wet clothing.

6. Keep the body warm, cover with blankets.

7. When the victim becomes conscious, give hot drinks.

8. Do not allow him to sit up.

9. After doing the above, remove quickly to hospital as a stretcher case.

STRANGULATION

Strangulation is, usually, the result of throttling by hands or a rope or scarf being tied round the neck.

Management

1. Cut or remove the band.

2. Give artificial respiration

3. Do the above immediately.

CHOKING

This is most common with children, a marble, a bead or a button may get struck in the air passage. In adults also the food may go down the wrong way and choke him. The aim of first aid is to remove the foreign body or obstruction.

Management in the case of an adult

When the victim is standing, the first aider should stand behind the victim and wrap his arms around the waist. Grasp the fist with your other hand and place the thumb of the fist against the abdomen, slightly above the naval and below the rib cage.

Press your fist into the victims abdomen with a quick upward thrust. Repeat several times, if necessary, till the foreign body is expelled out of the wind pipe. When the victim is sitting, the first aider stands behind

111

the chair and performs the same manoeuvre. If the victim is lying, turn him supine facing the victim, kneel astride like victims legs with your hands, one on top of another, place the heel of your bottom hand over the abdomen between the naval and rib cage. Press into the victims abdomen with a quick upward thrust, repeat several times. If necessary, should the patient vomit, place him on his side and wipe to prevent asphyxia. Following the expulsion of food particles foreign body, it may be necessary to give artificial respiration.

In the case of an infant

1. Hold him upside down by the legs and smack his back hard three or four times.

2. If it is not successful, lay the child prone position with his head hanging downwards over the knee and give sharp smacks between shoulders

3. If it is not successful, induce vomiting by passing two fingers right to the back of the throat.

Artificial respiration

There have been several methods of artificial respiration, practiced in first aid upto the II world war. Sylvester's method was felt to be the best. During the war, mouth to mouth method was discovered and found to be the best and easiest method to be used under most conditions.

Asphyxia of a severe degree is found along with unconsciousness. General causes are :-

a) The tongue may have fallen back into the throat

b) Vomit or spittle may have collected in the throat or

c) Some foreign material may have collected and obstructed the air passages.

Therefore, when a casualty is unconscious, make sure, he is breathing freely.

Begin to work immediately as every minute counts. Do not delay.

Treatment when not breathing

1. Loosen all clothing at waist, chest and neck.

2. Tilt the head backwards while supporting the back of neck with your palm. This will lift the tongue to its normal position. Thus, the air passage will be cleared and the casualty may begin to breathe after a gasp.

3. If breathing does not begin after the above treatment, help movements of chest and lungs, four or five times. This will be, usually, enough to start breathing. If breathing does not start even now, mouth to mouth breathing should be begun.

Mouth to Mouth

1. Place the casualty on his back. Hold his head tilted back.

2. Take a deep breath with mouth open widely.

3. Keep nostrils of casualty pinched.

4. Cover the mouth of the casualty with your mouth.

5. Watching the chest, blow into his lungs until the chest bellow up, withdraw your mouth, note the chest falls back.

6. Repeat the above 15 to 20 times a minute.

7. If casualty is young, the operations are as above but your open mouth should cover both the mouth and nose of the casualty and blow gently.

8. If the chest does not rise, look for an obstruction.

   a) Turn the casualty to a side and thump his back. This will make the obstructing material come to the front of the throat. Open the mouth and remove it with your fingers, covered with a piece of cloth.

b) If a child, hold it up by the feet and thump the back.

9. Use mouth-to-nose respiration if mouth-to-mouth is not possible, but note the casualty's mouth should be closed by the first aider's thumb.

10. If the heart is working, continue artificial respiration until normal breathing occurs.

Send for ambulance.

11. If the heart is not working, you will notice the following:

a) The face is blue or pale

b) Pupils are dilated

c) Heart beats and pulse at root of the neck are not to be felt.

Treatment

a) Place the casualty flat on his back on a hard surface.

b) Give a smart hit with the edge of your hand on the lower and left angle of the sternum. This, usually, stimulates the heart to work.

c) In case the heart does not work, persists the striking for 10-15 seconds, at the rate of one stroke a second. Feel for the pulse at the root of neck all the time. If the pulse becomes regular and continuous stop treating.

d) All the while, artificial respiration has to go on.

External heart compression

This method can be used if there are two trained persons.

114

a) This should go on along with artificial respiration. Therefore, ask the first aider giving mouth-to-mouth breathing to sit to the right of the casualty and place yourself on the left side.

b) Feel and mark the lower part of the sternum.

c) Place the heel of your hand on the marked part.

d) Place the heel of the other hand over it.

e) With your right arm, press the sternum backwards.

Important notes

a) Even if the casualty is breathing, but the breathing is not normal, it is wise to start artificial respiration.

b) Do not begin thumping the heart or compression until you are sure that the heart has stopped beating.

Strangulation and Hanging

Strangulation is, usually the result of throttling by hands or a rope or scarf being tied tightly round the neck.

In hanging the fracture of spine causing compression or tear of the spinal cord is more important.

Management

1. Cut or remove the band constricting the throat.

2. If suspended, raise the body and loosen or cut the rope.

3. Give artificial respiration

4. To do the above, do not wait to the policemen but inform the authorities later.

FROST BITE

Here, local tissues are frozen, usually at the extremities. They become injured by continuous constriction of the surface blood vessels, because of exposing to extreme cold. The damage may be superficial or deep.

The affected areas become, at first, pale, then waxy white and then blue colour and finally, black. Blistering may occur. The patient may complain of "pins and needles" and severe pain. Then the part becomes gradually numb and freezing bites deeper. The skin becomes hard and stiff.

The affected area may be warmed slowly and naturally to prevent further destruction. Take the patient to the hospital at the earliest. Do not rub the area. Do not burst the blisters. Do not heat the part with fires or hot water bottles. Do not allow the patient to smoke.

Handle the damaged tissues gently. Remove frozen coverings carefully. Warm the part with your own hands. Take the patient to warm surroundings as soon as possible. The patient may walk on frost-bitten feet before thawing out, but not after wards. Carry the patient on a stretcher. If the colour does not return quickly, the affected part may be kept in warm water. When the part thaws out the colour will improve and there will be pain. The thawed area may be dried and dressed with dry gauze or wool and bandage it lightly. Elevate the part to reduce swelling. On the advice of the doctor, give the patient two paracetamol tablets. Remove the patient to the hospital on a stretcher.

Heat exhaustion

This is caused by loss of salt and water from the body. It is more common in people, not accustomed to working in a very hot, humid environment.

The patient may feel exhausted but restless. The patient may have a headache and feel tired, dizzy and nauseated. Muscular cramps may occur in abdomen and lower limbs. Patient's face will be pale and skin will feel cold and clammy. Breathing becomes fast and shallow, pulse is rapid and weak. Temperature may remain normal or fall. The patient may faint by sudden movement.

Remove the patient to a cooler environment and replace lost fluids and minerals. Place the patient in a cool place. If he is conscious, give him sips of cold water to drink. If he is sweating profusely, has cramp, diarrhoea or vomiting add 1/2 a teaspoon of salt to each 1/2 litre of water. If the patient becomes unconscious, open his airway and check breathing. Complete the A B C of resuscitation, if necessary, and place him in the recovery position. Seek medical aid.

Sun burn

Serious discomfort and even, superficial burns may be caused by the direct rays of the sun and sometimes blisters may be caused. In hot countries even short

117

periods of exposure to midday sun can cause severe burns. Prevention is better than cure and so, people should be warned to take reasonable precautions. First aider is necessary as the symptoms of sun burn appear a few hours after it is caused. The patient should be advised to see a doctor unless the condition is obviously trivial. If necessary, general rules for the treatment of burns and scalds should be applied.

SHOCK

A condition of severe depression of the vital function is called shock. It is associated with changes in the circulatory system varying from temporary weakness to complete failure. Its severity depends on the nature and extent of the injury and a common cause of death after severe injuries.

Shock may develop immediately or after sometime. This delay may occur because the absence of signs and symptoms may give rise to a sense of false security or due to the injury being under estimated loss of entire blood or plasma from the circulation, is the prime cause of shock. Severe shock occurring immediately after most injuries other than burns, is almost always due to bleeding to the outside into the tissue or the body cavities. In the case of burns, there may be lot of plasma loosing into the tissues. Simple fracture of the femur may cause 20 to 30% loss of blood volume by concealed bleeding in the thigh. Compound fractures of tibia and fibula can cause 15-20% of the total volume of blood. On multiple injuries, each contributes its share of blood loss.

The severity of shock depends upon the amount and speed of the bleeding. In the beginning the circulatory system may be able to adapt itself to the loss of blood and continue to function more or less adequately. But the condition of the patient will become more and more critical as time passes, unless the bleeding is stopped and blood volume is restored by the blood transfusion.

Different kinds of shock

There are four types of shock

1. Nerve shock
2. Established shock
3. Hypovolaemic shock
4. Cardiogenic shock

Common signs and symptoms of shock

These may be for transient attack of faintness or a state of collapse and they are,-

1. Giddiness and faintness
2. Sudden fall of temperature
3. Nausea
4. Pallor
5. Cold clammy skin
6. A slow pulse at first and then becomes progressively more feeble and rapid.
7. Vomiting
8. Unconsciousness

1. Nerve Shock

All forms of shock involves some nervous reaction. But it is possible to deal separately by a type of shock which is caused entirely by nervous factors. It causes a fall in blood pressure but this need not be associated with any reduction in the volume of circulating blood.

2. Established shock

Patients with more than minor injuries, may develop a more serious condition called, established

119

shock. This may be expected when there are major injuries. But when the injuries are deep and bleeding is concealed, the condition of the patient is just as dangerous.

If there is failure of circulation, shock will increase and produce symptoms and signs of established shock. There are, as stated above, but more pronounced and the patients colour may become ash gray. Collapse will be more obvious and the pulse more feeble and respiration increases.

3. Hypovolaemic shock

Due to loss of body fluids commonly occurs in burns, Road traffic accidents etc.

4. Cardiogenic shock

Occurs due to sudden heart attack.

General treatment of shock

1. Reassure the patient

2. Lay him on his back with head low and turned to one side unless there is injury to the head, abdomen or chest when the shoulder must be raised and supported.

   If he has vomited or if there is interference with breathing, place him in the three quarter prone position.

3. Loosen clothing about the neck, chest and waist.

4. Wrap him in a blanket or rug.

5. If he complains of thirst, give him sips of water.

6. Do not apply heat or friction to the limbs. Hot water bottles should not be used.

120

Special treatment for established shock:-
Proceed as described above. Bear in mind that, in severe cases transfusion and surgery are matters of grave urgency if you want to save life. So, it is unwise to delay transfer to hospital, for, as long as even five minutes, except to deal with falling respiration, to stop severe bleeding, to dressing a sucking wound of the chest or to secure a limb badly broken.

7. Do not give anything by mouth (the patient may require anaesthesia).

8. Tilt the stretcher in such a way as to lower the level of the head from the rest of the body except in cases of head, chest or abdominal injury.

9. Remove urgently to hospital.

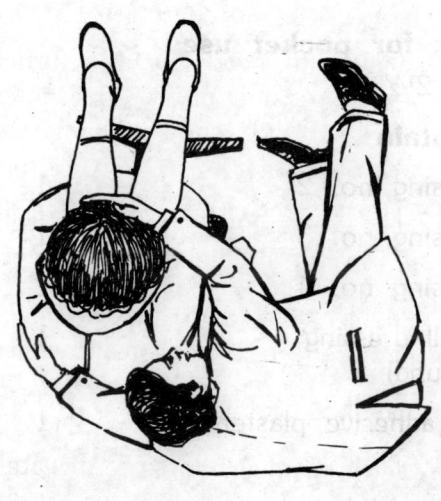

FIRST AID PROCEDURE
SUPPLIES AND EQUIPMENTS

First aid appliances should be kept in a metal or plastic box which can be opened and closed easily. The box should be labelled clearly and Red cross sign and "First Aid" should be written on it. The box should be kept away from children. As and when the items are consumed, they should immediately replaced.

Small first aid box for pocket use
    6" X 3½" X 2½"

It should contain

1.	First aid dressing no. 2	-	1
2.	First aid dressing no. 3	-	1
3.	First aid dressing no. 4	-	1
4.	Sterilized small dressing (for burnt wound)	-	1
5.	Small roll of adhesive plaster 1/2" X 1 m	-	1
6.	Soframycin skin ointment	-	1
7.	Safety pins (6 packets)	-	1

8.	Roller bandages 1"	-	1
9.	Cotton wool small pocket	-	1
10.	Eye pad	-	1
11.	Small scissors	-	1
12.	Small forceps	-	1

Large Fist aid box used to in big Institutions and Factories

17½" X 10" X 6½" It is a dirt proof box.

It may contain

1.	First aid book	1
2.	Sterilized dressing no. 18 for fingers 12	
3.	Sterilized dressing no. 24 for hands and feet	12
4.	Big sterilized dressing no. 20	12
5.	Dressing for burnt wound	

	Big	2
	Medium	4
	Small	6

6.	Sterilized cotton wool (25 gms)	6 pkts
7.	Soframycin ointment	2 tubes
8.	Savlon or Dettol antiseptic solution	2 bottles
9.	Chloromycetin eye ointment	2 t..
10.	Eye pad 6	
11.	Adhesive plaster (big)	1
12.	Roller bandage -	

	2.5 cm X 5 cm	6
	5 cm X 5 cm	6
	7.5 cm X 5 cm	6

123

13. Triangular bandage   12
14. Safety pin (10 Nos.)   1 pkt
15. Scissors 12.7 cm (end pointed)   1
16. Cotton wool for pad (50 gms)   2 pkts
17. Gauze cloth 28" X 8" in
    pressed pack   1. pkt
18. Aspirin (300 mg) tablets (24 tabs)   1 bottle
19. Adhesive dressing strip (band aid)   10
20. Big sized torch   1
21. Pad and pencil for writing
    writing card   1

Medium First aid box
Contents

1. One set first aid splints wooden.
2. 12 Triangular bandages.
3. 3 Packets sterilized cotton wool (25 Grams).
4. 6 First aid dressing (3 large and 3 medium)
5. 9 Roller bandages assorted.
6. 3 Burn dressings assorted
7. 2 Eye pads.
8. 1 Packet of safety pin (10 Nos).
9. One scissor ordinary 12.7 cms.
10. One roll adhesive plaster.
11. 1 Tube cetavlon.
12. 1 Bottle dettol antiseptic.
13. 1 Tube eye ointment of sulphacetamide
    preparation.

124

14. Loose woven gauze in a compressed pack.

15. 1 Bottle aspirin (300 Mg 124 Tablets).

16. 1 Tear off scribbling pad with a pencil and a pen in plastic cover.

17. 10 Adhesive dressing strips.

18. 1 Record card in plastic cover.

19. 2 Feet dressing of the modified armp.

20. One torch medium size of Eveready (with cells).

BANDAGES AND SLINGS

Applications of bandages

These are made from flannel, calico elastic net or special paper, they can be improvised by any of the above material, one from stockings or ties.

Bandages are used to

Maintain direct pressure over a dressing to control bleeding.

Retain dressing and slings in position.

Prevent or reduce swelling.

Provide support for a limb or joint.

Restrict movement.

Assets in lifting and carrying casualty.

Bandages should be applied firm enough to keep dressing and splints in position. But not so tight as to cause injury to the part or to impede the circulation of the blood. A bluish tinge of the finger or nails may be a danger sign that the bandages are too tight. Loss of sensation is an other sign.

125

Types of bandages

1. Triangular.
2. Roller.
3. Special-such as, many tail or 'T' bandages.

Triangular bandage

The triangular bandage may be used in nursing and for slings, to support an arm after injury.

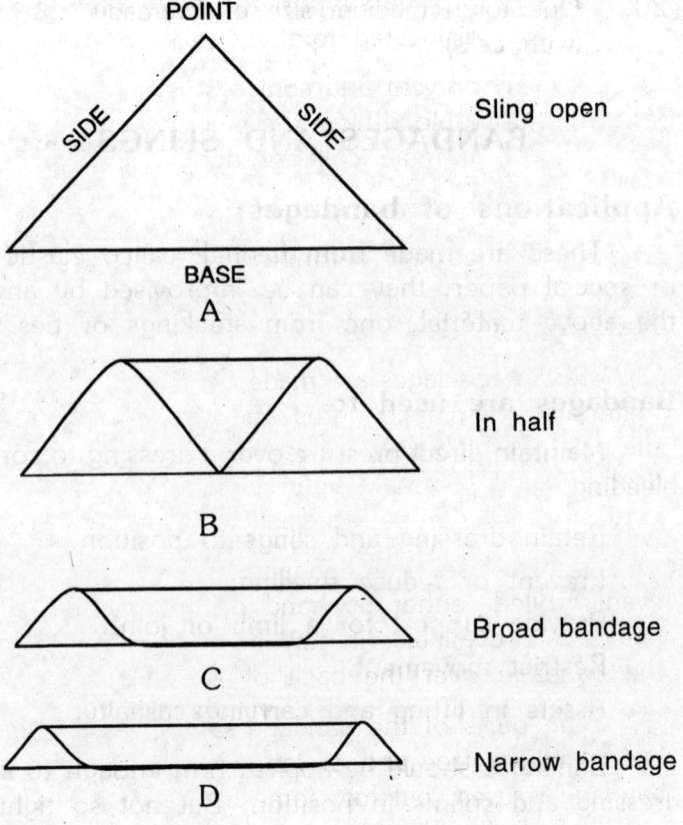

Figure 45. Triangular bandage

Roller bandages

Uses

Roller bandages are used for the following purposes.

1. To cover and to retain dressing and splints in position.
2. To exercise pressure on a part in order to prevent or to reduce swelling.
3. To provide support for a part, as a sprained or dislocated joint.
4. To prevent and control haemorrhage, and to drive blood from the part, bandaged, in cases of extreme collapse due to haemorrhage.
5. To restrict movement.
6. To correct deformity.

Materials

Roller bandages are made from strips of different material of varying lengths and widths, according to the part to which they are applied. Materials commonly used include, flannel, open wove cotton, fast edge cotton, calico, crepe or elastic net.

Before use, the bandage should be firmly and evenly rolled, either by hand or by machine. If two people are available, it may be found helpful to run the bandage over the back of a chair.

The parts of the bandage are referred to as the head and the free end or tail. Usually, a single roller bandage is used, but for, some certain parts, a double headed roller bandage is required. In this, the free ends of two roller bandages are sew together leaving the heads to close together, on the same side of the bandage.

Most roller bandages are 6 yards long, except the very narrow ones, which are, usually, short. The width lay according to the part of the body to be bandaged. The usual width of the bandages are, 1 Inch to 4 to 6 inches.

Part bandage	Width
Fingers	1 inch.
Arm	2 to 2 inches.
Leg	3 to 3 inches.
Trunk	4 to 6 inches.
Head	2 inches.

Rules for the application of roller bandages

1. Use a tightly rolled bandage of the correct width.

2. Support the part to be bandaged through out, for the forearm, the hand should be prone.

3. Always stand in front of the patient, except, when applying a cape line bandage.

4. Bandage a limb in the position in which it is to remain.

5. Hold the bandage with the head uppermost and apply the outer surface of the bandage to the part, never unroll more than a few inches of bandage at a time.

6. Bandage from within outwards and from below upwards, maintaining even pressure throughout.

7. Begin the bandage with a firm oblique turn to fix it and allow each successive turn to cover two thirds of the previous one, with the free edges lying parallel.

8. Make any reverses or crossing a line on the outer side of the limb, except, when this brings them over a wound or prominence of bone, in which case, they must be on the front of the limb.

9. Pad the axilla or groin when bandaging these parts, so that, two of the surfaces of skin do not touch beneath the bandage.

10. Finish off with a straight turn above the part, hold in the end and fasten with a safety pin.

Points to be observed

1. The comfort of the patient is the first consideration, except, when arresting haemorrhage or correcting a deformity.

2. Neatness and economy must be considered, but, the bandages must fulfill its purpose and must cover the dressing completely.

3. The bandage should be firm and applied with even pressure throughout, but the extremities must be carefully watched for any signs of swelling or blueness due to interference with circulation by a bandage that is too light.

Turns used in roller bandaging

1. Simple spiral
2. Reverse spiral
3. Figure of eight
4. Spica

Simple spiral

Is used for parts which are of uniform thickness, such as, a finger, a wrist. The bandage is applied obliquely round the part, each turn cover two thirds (2/3) of the proceeding one, and the edges being kept parallel.

129

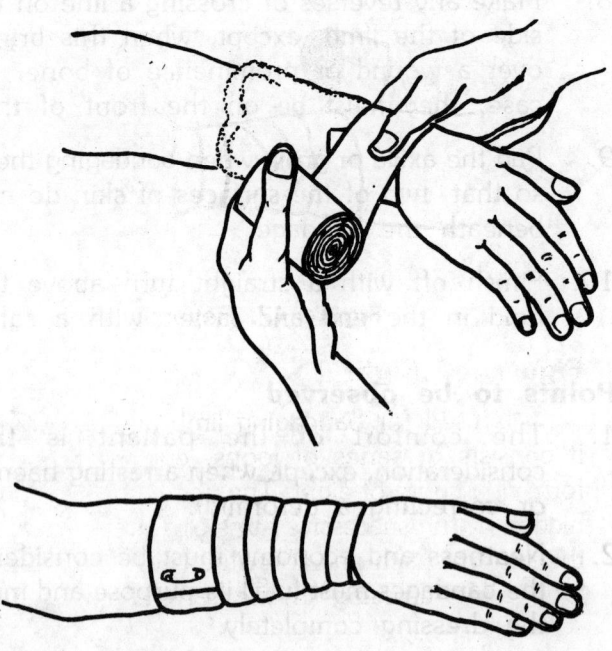

Figure 46. Simple Spiral

Reverse spiral

It is used for parts which vary in thickness and upon which the bandage of circular turns cannot be tied properly like leg and forearms. One or two simple spiral turns are usually made to carry the bandages to the point at which the spiral can no longer be employed, and then the lower edge of its last spiral is fixed with the thumb about halfway between the mid line and outer surface of the limb. The bandage is then reversed and brought down and carried round the limb, when another reverse is made immediately above the former one. These reverses are repeated as far as necessary and the bandage completed with one or two spiral turns straight round the limb. Care should be taken and that, each reverse occurs immediately above the previous one, so that, the pattern is even. Each turn should cover two thirds of the preceding one, as in the simple spiral.

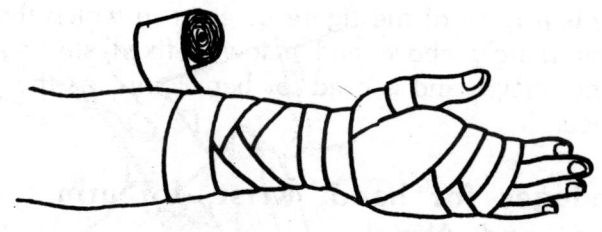

Figure 47. Reverse spiral

Figure of Eight

Is used for bandaging limb and for covering joints. It consists of series of loops, encircling the part in the form of a figure of eight. The upper loops being completely hidden by the successive turns end the lower loops forming the pattern. Each one cover the two thirds of the preceding loop and crossing in the same line.

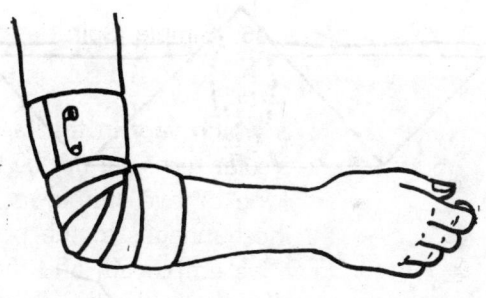

Figure 48. Figure of Eight bandage

The Spica

Is a form of the figure of eight in which one turn is very much larger than the other. It is used for joints at right angles to the body. Eg: Shoulder, Groin and Thumb.

131

The Divergent Spica

Is a form of the figure of eight in which the turn go alternately above and below a fixed starting turn ending above, and is used for bent joints, as the elbow or heel.

Bandages for hand, wrist, forearm, elbow and Arm

Hand Bandage

With the pronated, that is, the palm held down wards fix the bandage by a turning round the wrist and carry the roll obliquely over the back of the hand to the side of the little finger. Carry the bandage round the palm, encircling the finger with one horizontal turn,

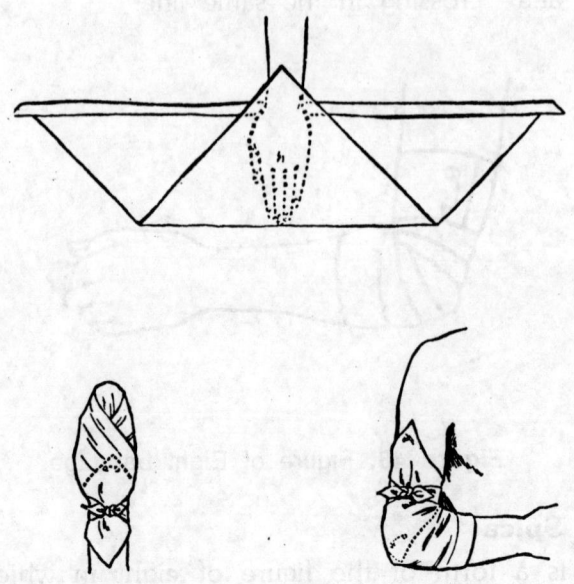

Figure 49. Hand bandage (when the injury is on the palm)

so that the lower boarder of the bandage, just touches the root of the nail of the little finger. Carry the bandage one more round the palm and then return obliquely to the wrist. The figure of eight turn round the wrist and hand are repeated until the hand is covered and the bandage is then finished with a spiral turn round the wrist.

Wrist, Forearm, and Upper arm Bandages

The wrist and forearm are bandaged by use of the simple and reverse spiral until the elbow is reached. The figure of eight turn can be so used, as the limb enlarges as an alternative to the reverse spiral turn, if preferred.

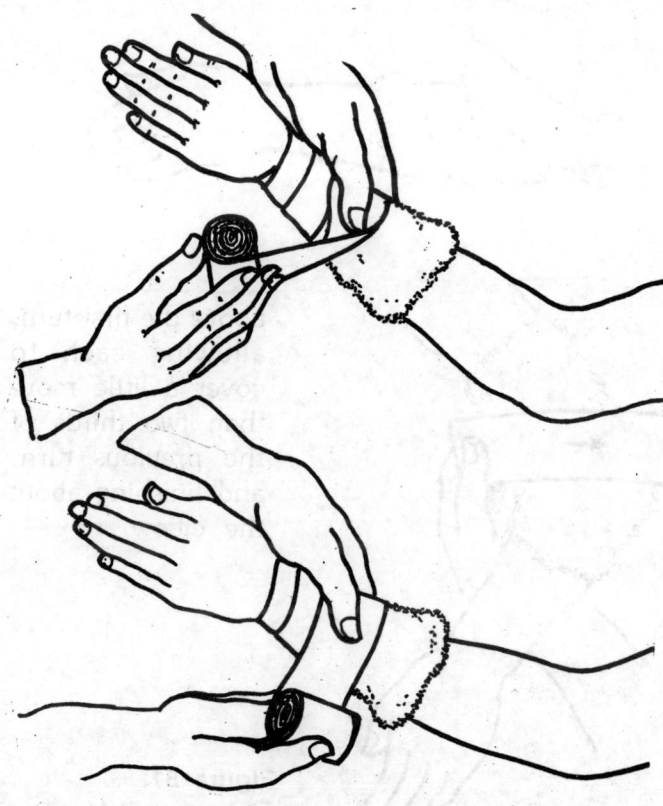

Figure 50. Wrist bandage

To Cover the elbow

Bend the elbow at right angles, lay the outer side of the bandage on the inner side of the joint and take one straight turn carrying the bandage over the elbow tip and round the limb of the elbow. The second turn is made to encircle forearm and the third arm. Each of these turns being made to cover the margins of the first turn. Continue the turns alternately, below and

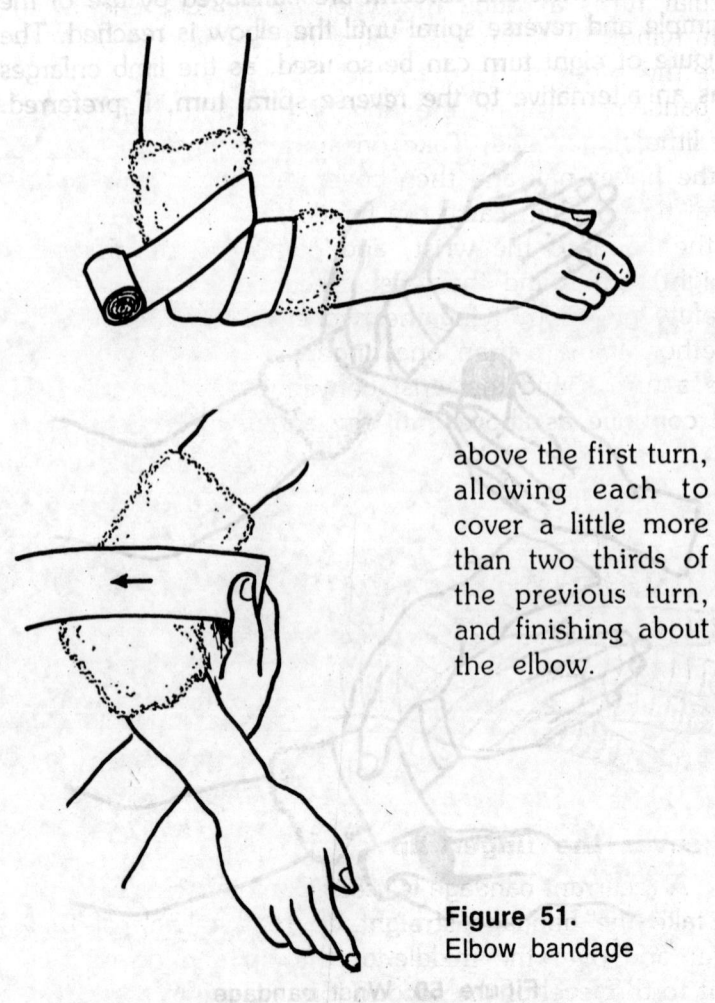

above the first turn, allowing each to cover a little more than two thirds of the previous turn, and finishing about the elbow.

Figure 51.
Elbow bandage

134

The Upper Arm

The bandages, as is the forearm, by a succession of reverse spirals or figure of eight turns, and the bandages may be carried on from the forearm, or elbow or started independently, as most conveniently.

Finger Bandages

With the hand pronated, fix the bandage by two circular turns a round the wrist leaving the end free from tying off. Afterwards, carry the bandage obliquely over the back of hand to the base of the finger to be bandaged. Taking the fingers is order, start from the little finger side. Take on spiral turn to the base of the finger nail and then cover the finger by simple spiral turns. Then carry the bandage a cross the back of the hand to the wrist, and complete it with one straight turn round the wrist. Secure th₂ bandage by a safety pin or by tying the two ends of the bandage together. If more than one finger as to be bandaged, take a turn round the wrist between each two fingers and continue as above until the bandage is complete.

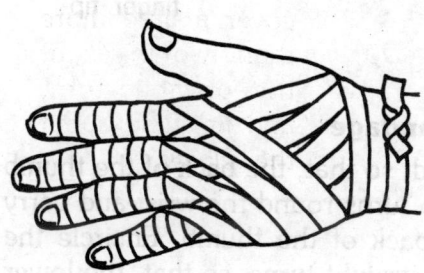

Figure 52.
Finger bandages

To cover the finger tip

A recurrent bandage is used. Commence as before, but take the bandage straight up to the back of the finger and over the middle of the tip and down the front to the level of the second joint. Holding the turns

135

back and front with the fingers of the other hand, make two more turns over the tip of the finger, one on either side of the first turn. Fix the loop with a straight circular turn as near to the tip as possible and then cover the finger by simple spiral turns as before. Being careful to make them from within outwards. Take a straight turn round the wrist and either finish off as before or continue the next finger.

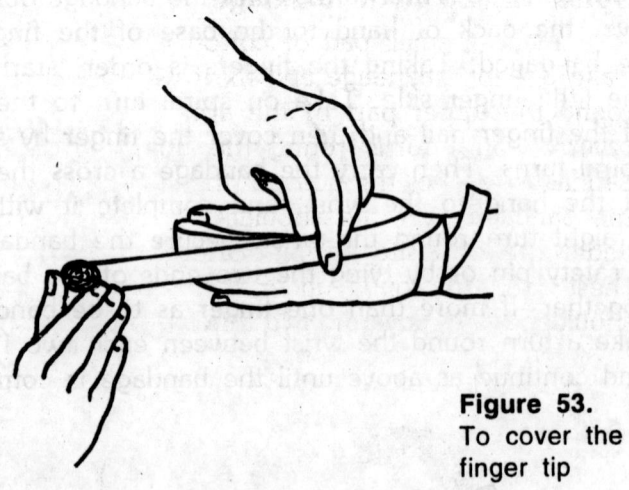

Figure 53.
To cover the finger tip

Spica of Thumb Bandage

With the hand held, so that, the back of the thumb is upper most, take two turns round the wrist and carry the bandage over the back of the thumb. Encircle the thumb with one or two straight turns, so that, the lower border of the bandage is level with the root of the nail. Carry the bandage back, over the back of the hand, round the wrist and repeat the figure of eight turns round thumb and wrist, until the wall of the thumb is completely covered. Complete the bandages with one straight turn, round the wrist.

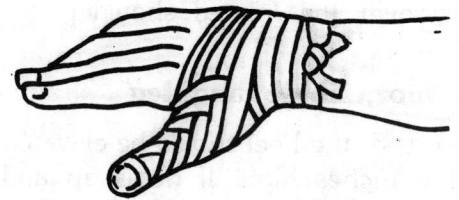

Figure 54.
Thumb
bandage

Spica of shoulder bandage

Place a small pad of cotton wool in each axilla.
Take 3-4 inch bandage and fix it with two spiral turns
round the upper part of the arm. Take two or three
reverse spiral turns round the upper arm until the
bandages reaches the point of the shoulder. Then carry
the bandage over the shoulder, across the back and
under the opposite armpit. Bring it back across the
chest and arm round under the armpit and over the
shoulder again, covering two thirds of the previous turn.

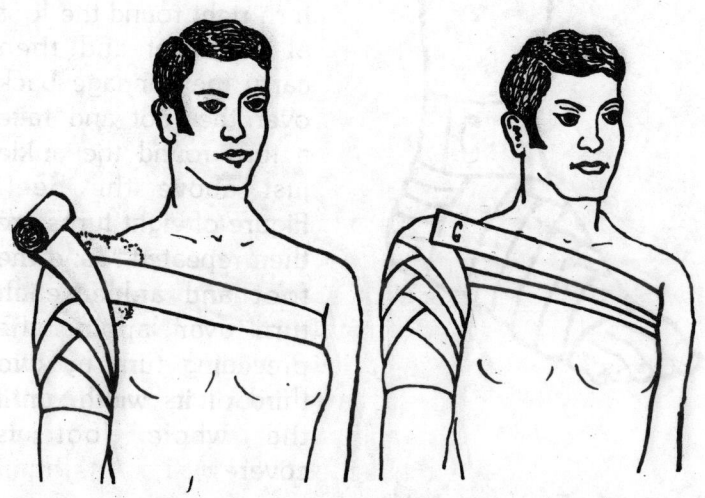

Figure 55. Shoulder bandage

137

This forms a figure of eight round the arm and the body and the turns are repeated until the whole shoulder is covered. The bandage should be secured by a pin immediately over the injured shoulder.

Bandages for the foot, ankle and leg

If the patient is in bed, the heel should be elevated on a support, about 6 inches high. If he is up and about, he should be seated in a chair with the foot supported on a stool or another chair. To avoid stooping, the nurse may, if she prefers, sit opposite to the patient and take his foot on her knee.

Foot and ankle bandage

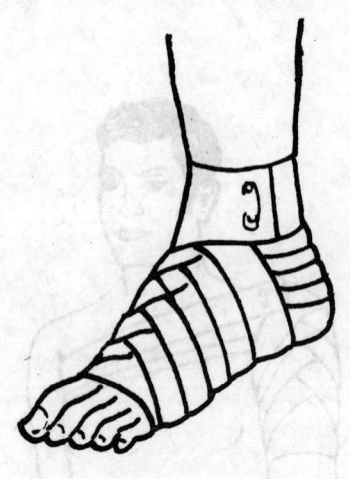

Take one or two turns round the ankle to fix the bandage and then take it on obliquely across the foot to the root of the little toe. Make one horizontal turn right round the foot at his level and then carry the bandage back over the foot and take a turn round the ankle just above the heel. Figure of eight turns are then repeated round the foot and ankle, each turn over lapping the preceding turn by two third of its width, until the whole foot is covere

Figure 56. Foot and Ankle bandage

138

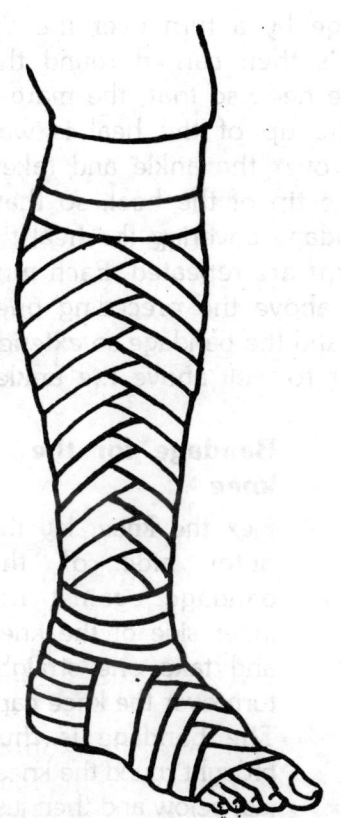

Leg

If the bandage is to be continued up the leg, the reverse spiral or figure of eight turns may be used as for the arm.

Figure 57. Leg bandage

To cover the heel

The leg should be supported, so that, the heel projects well over the edge of the chair, stool or cushion on which it is placed.

The foot should be kept at right angles to the leg.

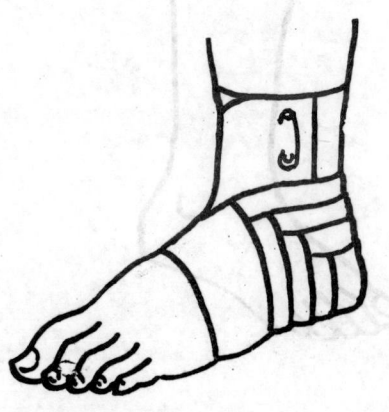

Figure 58. Heel bandage

Commence the bandage by a turn over the tip of the heel. The bandage is then carried round the foot just below the tip of the heel, so that, the margin of the bandage covering the tip of the heal is well covered. It is then brought over the ankle and taken round the leg, just above the tip of the heel, so that, the other margin of the bandage covering the heel tip is now also covered. The turns are repeated. Each turn being made just below and above the preceding one, until the heel is well covered and the bandage so extends from halfway along the foot to well above the ankle.

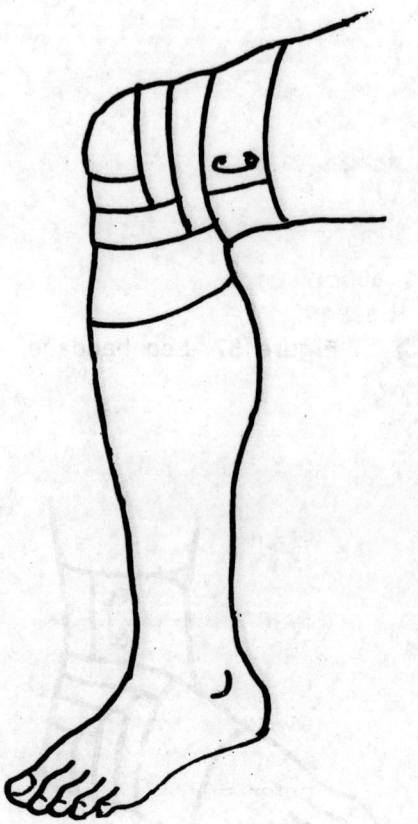

Bandage for the knee

Flex the knee, lay the outer side of the bandage against the inner side of the knee and take one straight turn over the knee cap. The bandage is thus brought round the knee, just below and then just above. Note that the margins of the bandage covering the knee cap are covered as in the elbow and heel bandages. The turns are repeated below and above the joint until the whole knee is covered and the bandage is then secured by one straight turn round the thigh.

Figure 59. Knee bandage

Spica of hip bandage

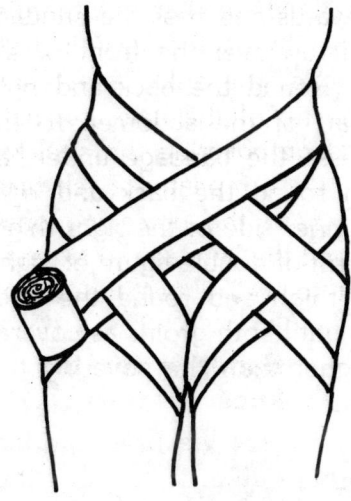

Figure 60. Hip bandage

Place the outside of the bandage on the inner side of the thigh about 6 inches below the groin. Carry the bandage horizontally round the limb and make three or four ascending reverse spiral turns round the thigh. Carry the bandages from within outwards over the front of the groin and up round the hip and back, passing over the prominence of the hip bone on the opposite side. Bring the bandage down, over the abdomen to the outer side of the thigh and repeat the figure of eight round the body and the thigh until the hip is covered.

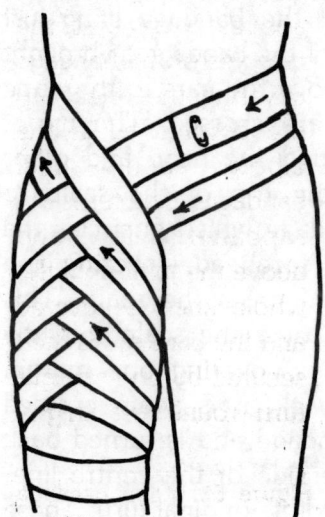

Spica of groin bandage

This is applied in the same way as the spica for the hip, except that the bandage is started higher up. The reverse spiral and omitted and the crossings are made over the front of the groin instead of on the outer side of the front of the thigh.

Figure 61. Groin bandage

141

Double spica of groin bandage

Lay the outer surface of the bandage over the right groin from without inwards and pass the bandage round the thigh, carrying it up over the front of the right groin to the left hip. Round the back and right hip and over the lower part of the abdomen to the outer side of the thigh. Pass the bandage under the thigh, up to the left groin round the back and right hip and down again to the inner side of the right thigh. These turns, which really form of double figure of eight, round the body and right thigh and round the body and left thigh, are repeated until both groins as covered each turn being slightly higher than the covering two thirds of the preceding one.

Head and other bandage

Capeline bandage

This bandage is, sometimes, used when the whole scalp is to be covered. A double headed roller bandage is used. The patient should be seated and the nurse should stand behind the patient. Place the centre of the outer surface of the bandage in the centre of the forehead, the lower border of the bandage lying just above the eyebrows. The head of the bandage as brought round over the temples and above the ears to the nape of the neck where the ends are crossed. The upper bandage being carried on, round the head and other brought over the centre of the top of the scalp to the root of the nose. The bandage which encircles the head is now brought over the forehead, covering and fixing the bandage which could cross the scalp. This bandage is then brought back over the scalp. Slightly to one side of the centre, thus covering one margin of the original turn. At the back, it is again crossed and fixed by the encircling bandage and is turned back over the scalp to the opposite side of the centre line, now covering the other margin of its original turn. These backward and forward turns are repeated to alternate side of the centre, each one being, in turn, fixed by the encircling bandage until the whole scalp is covered. The bandages is completed by a circular turn round the head and pinned in the centre of the forehead.

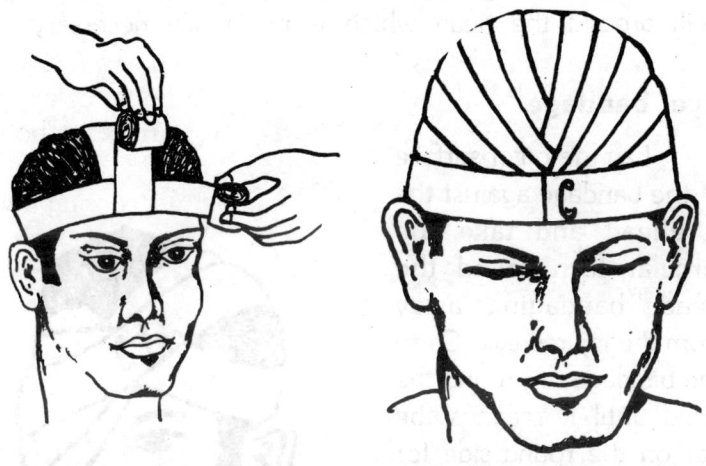

Figure 62. Capeline bandages

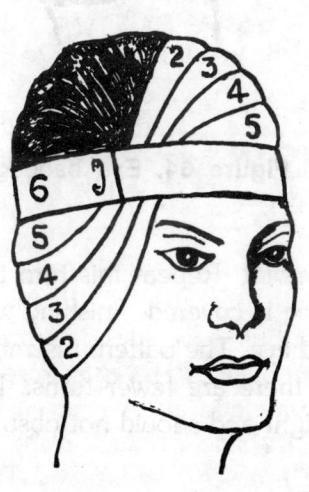

Ear bandage

Lay the outer surface of the bandage against the forehead and carry the bandage round the head in one circular turn, bandaging away from the injured ear. Towards the sound side, carry the bandage round to the back of the head, low down in the nape of the neck again, repeat these.

Figure 63. Ear bandage

143

Each turn being slightly higher than the previous one as it cover the dressing, but slightly lower as it covers the hair. Continue until the whole is covered and complete the bandage by one straight turn around the forehead, pinning where all the turns cross one another. Some people prefer to take the bandage round the forehead between each turn covering the dressing, but this makes a heavy bulk around the head which is not really necessary.

Eye bandage

Lay the outer surface of the bandage against the forehead and take the circular turn round the head, bandaging away from the injured eye. Carry the bandage on, round the head until it reaches the ear on the round side for the second time. Take it obliquely to the back of the head, under the prominence at the back of the skull and from there bring it upwards beneath the ear of the affected side, over the pad of the eye to the circular turn and continue

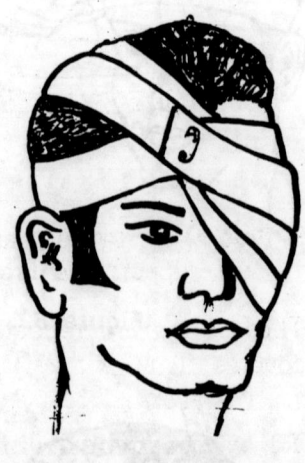

Figure 64. Eye bandage

over the head to the starting point. Repeat this turn two or three times until the dressing is covered, finishing with a safety pin just above the good eye. The pattern resembles that of the ear bandage, but there are fewer turns. The bandage should be light in weight and should not obstruct the view of the good eye.

144

Breast bandages to support one breast

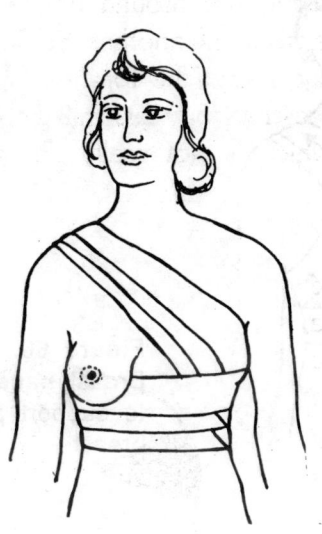

Figure 65. Breast bandage to support one breast

Take a 3 inch bandage and starting below the breast to be covered and working away from it towards the sound side, carry the bandage twice round the waist. Bring the bandage up, under the breast to be supported over the opposite shoulder obliquely down across the back or under the arm and once more round the waist, on covering two third of the previous turns.

These turns are repeated until the breast is sufficiently covered.

To support both breasts

Start with two circular turns round the waist as for the single breast, starting under the right breast and bring the bandage up, under the right breast, over the left shoulder, obliquely down across the back, under the right arm and across the front of the waist, horizontally. Carry the bandage under the left arm, up across the back to the right shoulder and down across the chest, under the left breast. From here, it is passed under the left arm and turns horizontally across the back to beneath the right breast again. These turns are repeated until both breast are covered.

145

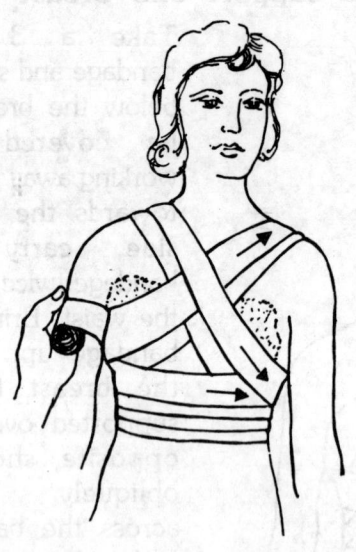

Figure 66.
Breast bandage
to support both
breasts

Stump bandage

Using a 4 inch bandage, place the end of the bandage in the centre of the upper side of the limb and carry the bandage, over the centre of the stump to the same level behind, holding the turns back and front with the thumb and fingers of the other hand. Repeat the recurrent turns over the end of the stump first and on the stump on the left and on the right side of the original turn

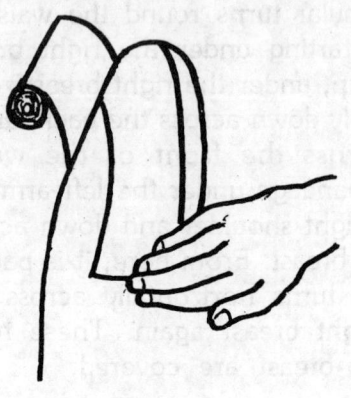

until the whole of the dressing is covered. Fix the loops with a straight turn around the stump until the dressing is completely covered and secure it with a safety pin. In an amputation of the leg above

146

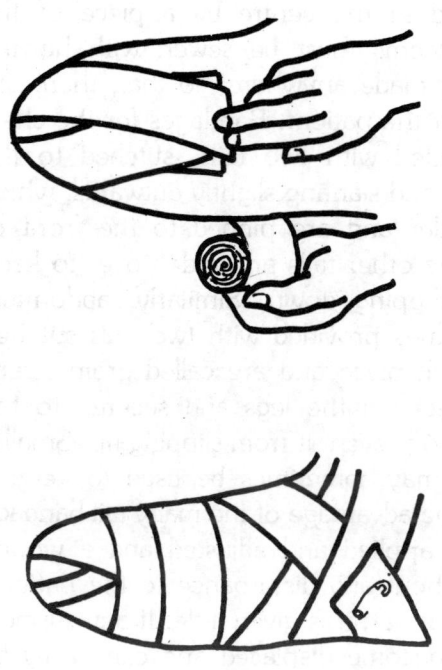

the knee, special care in bandaging is necessary to produce stump upon such an artificial limb can be worn on. To do this as soon as the dressing has been removed, a 6 inch crepe bandage should be applied firmly from below upward. The pressure around the stumps is gradually eased as the bandage is carried upwards as high as possible. The object being

Figure 67. Stump bandage

to produce a conical stump owing to stretching. The bandage may require re-application several times daily and the patient should never be allowed to go about on crutches when such a bandage is worn.

Special bandages

Many tail bandages

Many tail bandages are used for abdominal wound, certain chest dressing and for any part where the use of a roller bandage would entail a great amount of movement and exertion for the patient. It consists of a number of strips or tails of flannel domette or cotton material, 4-6 inches wide and of sufficient length to encircle the part and overlap atleast 8 inches. Each strip overlies the one above by two thirds of its width and the whole is secured in the centre by a piece of the same material. All seems must be sewen with herring bone and no turning made anywhere, so that, there are no hard ridges to hurt the patient. Bandages for the chest are sometimes provided with two tails, stitched to the top of the back piece and slanting slightly outwards, which pass over the shoulder and are pinned to the front of the bandage when the other tails are folded over to keep the bandage from slipping down. Similarly, abdominal bandages are sometimes provided with two tails stitched to the bottom of back piece and are called groin straps which are passed between the legs and secured to the front of the bandage to prevent it from slipping up. Smaller many tail bandages may sometimes be used to keep a dressing on a limb. The advantage of the many tail bandage are that, it is easily applied and adjusted and a wound can be inspected without any disturbance to the patient. The disadvantages are that, it is given little. If any support it tends to slip and become displaced and can easily be undone by the 'patient.

The application of an abdominal many tail bandage

For the bandage to be comfortably and efficiently applied, two people are required, although in an emergency one can manage. The patient should be lying quite flat before any attempts is made to apply or adjust a many tail bandage. The bandage is prepared with the tails rolled into the centre, from either end, the smooth portion of the back being uppermost and being placed next to the patient. The bandage is placed in the position, so that, the centre band lies under the patients back. The bandage is applied from below upwards. One tail being brought across the body at a time and held in position by a tail from the opposite side. The last tail is brought obliquely downwards and secured with a safety pin.

148

"T" bandages

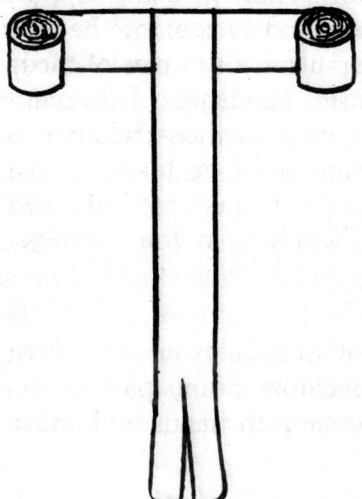

"T" bandages consist of two strips of flannel, about 4 inches wide, stitches together in the form of a "T". The horizontal strip is made long enough to pass round the body and the vertical strip is passed up between the legs. It is then pinned to the horizontal strip to keep rectal of perineal dressing in position.

Figure 68. "T" Bandage

Plaster of Paris bandages

Plaster bandages may be brought ready-made, such as, the "Gypsona" tape bandage or may be prepared by rubbing dry plaster of Paris into the meshes of strips of book muslin. Plaster of Paris bandages are used,

a) To make splints to immobilise fractures.

b) To protect the wound or to immobilize a part to relieve a pain and promote healing.

c) To make plaster beds and jackets.

The bandages are applied wet and as they dry, they form a hard protective covering. They take some time to dry and must be protected from bending or cracking until completely dry and set. A plaster tends to shrink as it dries and if it gets too light, it may impede circulation. A patient with a plaster applied to a limb should be instructed to report back to the hospital immediately if the extremely becomes blue, cc'l, or swollen.

149

Adhesive bandage

In certain circumstances, the doctor may order an adhesive bandage to be worn. These give fine support and may be used for protection and to promote healing in condition. Such as, varicose ulcer. Examples of those are elastoplast and viscopaste bandages. These are supplied according to similar rules to those relating to roller bandages. But great care must be taken to see that the bandage lies smoothly against the skin and that, there are no folds or wrinkles in the bandage.

Tubular gauze bandage

This is a special form of tubular bandage, which can be applied with an applicator to any part of the body. It is ideal for small dressing on hands and limbs.

Bandage for the jaw

Take a narrow strip of material, about 4 feet long or a narrow fold triangular bandage and place the centre of it, under the chin. Carry one end upwards over the top of the head and cross with the other end above the ear. Carry the shorter end low down across the front of the forehead and the larger end in to opposite direction round the back of the head and tie off close, above the other ear.

SLINGS

Uses of slings

1. To support injured arms.
2. To prevent pull by upper limb of injuries to chest, shoulder and the neck.

Different types of slings:

The arm slings

The arm sling is used in cases of fractured ribs, injuries of upper limbs and in cases of fracture in the

150

fore arm, wrist and hands after the application of splints or plaster casts and bandaging.

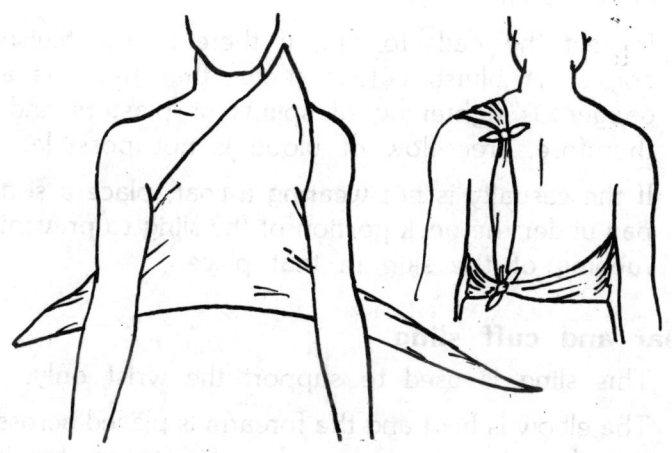

Figure 69. Arm sling

Applying the sling

1. Face the casualty, put one end of the spread triangular bandage over the uninjured shoulder with the point on the injured side.

2. Pass the end around the neck and bring it over the injured shoulder. The other end will, now, be hanging down over the chest.

3. Place the forearm horizontally across the chest and bring the hanging end up. The forearm is now covered by the bandage.

4. Tie the two ends in such a way that the forearm is horizontally or slightly tilted upwards and the knot is placed in the pit, above the collar bone.

5. Tuck the part of sling which is loose at the elbow, behind the elbow and bring the fold to the front and pin it up to the front of the bandage.

151

6. Place the tree base of the bandage in such a way that its margin is just at the base of the nail of the little finger. The nails of all the finger should be exposed.

7. Inspect the nails to see, if there is any bluish colour. A bluish colour shows that there is a dangerous tightening of splints or plasters and, therefore, free flow of blood is not possible.

8. If the casualty is not wearing a coat, place a soft pad under the neck portion of the sling to prevent rubbing of the skin in that place.

Collar and cuff sling

This sling is used to support the wrist only.

1. The elbow is bent and the forearm is placed across the chest in such a way that the fingers touch the opposite shoulder. In this position, the sling is applied.

2. A clove hitch is passed round the wrist and the ends tied in the hollow above the collar bone on the injured side.

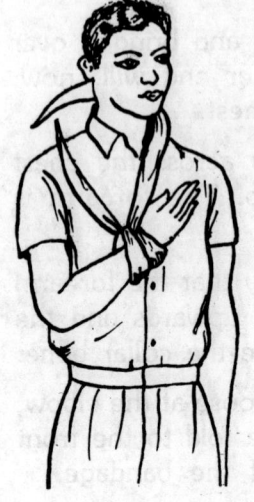 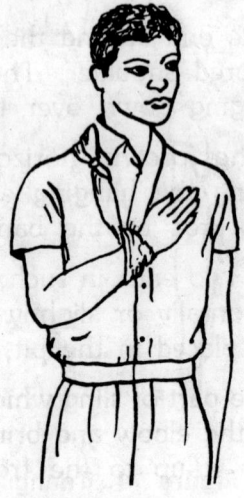

Figure 70.
Coller and
Cuff sling

152

Triangular sling

A triangular sling is used in treating a fracture of the collar bone. It helps to keep the hand raised high up, giving relief from pain due to the fracture.

1. Place the forearm across the chest with the fingers pointing towards the opposite shoulder and the palm over the breast bone.

2. Place an open bandage over the chest, with one end over the hand and the point beyond the elbow.

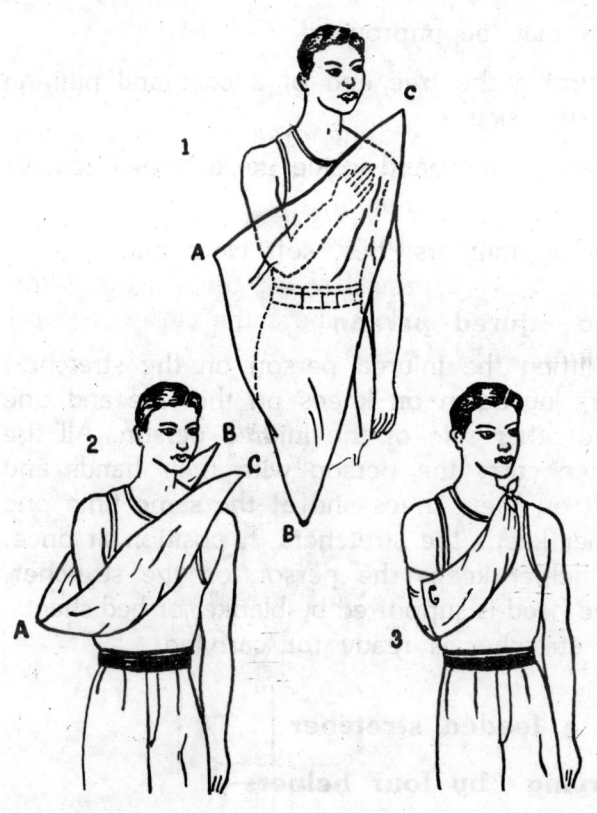

Figure 71. Triangular sling

153

3. Tuck the base of the bandage comfortably, under the forearm and hand.

4. Fold the lower end, also round the elbow and take it up and cross the back over the uninjured shoulder and tie it with the other free hand into the hollow, above the collar bone.

5. Tuck the point between forearm and bandage.

6. Tuck the fold, so formed, backwards over the lower half of the arm and fix it with a safety pin.

Improvised slings

Slings may be improvised.

1. By turning the free end of a coat and pinning it to the sleeve.

2. By passing the hand inside the buttoned coat or shirt.

3. By using mufflers, ties, soft cloth etc.,

Lifting an injured person

For lifting the injured person on the stretcher, the helpers lay down on knees on the side and one sits on the other side of the injured person. All the helpers then carry the person with their hands and so support on their knees and at the same time one other helper keeps the stretchers in position at once. Now the helper keeps the person on the stretcher, slowly. The head is supported by blanket or bed sheets. Now, the stretcher is ready for carrying.

Carrying a loaded stretcher

1. Carrying by four helpers

On indication from one helper, the other helpers lift the stretcher with their inner hand up to the length of their arms. All the four helpers proceed stepping first with their inner legs. These helpers should walk comfortably. If the helpers become tired, then the hand can be kept in comfortable position on the instruction of the other helper. Remember, do not carry the stretcher with the other hand while keeping the stretcher, gradually bending yourselves. On the instruction of one of the helper and all other helpers stand up, at the same time.

2. Carrying by two helpers

One helper stands towards the head end and one stands towards the foot end. Now both the helpers stand in between the two handles of the stretcher towards the hand feet side and on the instruction of one, both the helpers lift the stretcher up to the height of their limbs. Now on the instructions of one helper, both the helpers start walking. When the hand becomes tired, both the helpers can turn their hands and can keep them in comfortable position. While keeping the stretcher down, both the helpers bend down and slowly keep the stretcher. After keeping the stretcher on the ground, both the helpers stand up at the same time.

Unloading the stretcher

The injured person is unloaded from the stretcher after being brought to the hospital or house. The methods applied for the unloading are same as loading patient on the stretcher described earlier. If the injured person is lying in bedsheet or blanket, then he is picked up by the four corners with the help of four persons and is made to lie on the bed, then the sheet is drawn out. If the person is not lying on the blanket, then the helpers sit around the person in all sides, then they rest their hands below the head, waist, chest, hips and legs of the injured person and lift him up from the stretcher.

155

Rules for carrying casualties on stretchers:

1. Principally, the feet of the injured person should be in front side, when he is carried on a stretcher. But, in some cases where the stretcher is carried at height, on stairs or while coming down stairs, or if the leg is injured, the above rule is to be followed.

2. While walking on an uneven ground, the stretcher should be carried by four helpers wherever possible, the person should be carried on the even surface.

3. While crossing a ditch, the front helper should keep the stretcher on the back and then get down. Then they carry the stretcher for a while. The back portion of the stretcher is kept on the back and the helpers get down and then all the helpers walk forward. After crossing the front, the helpers keep the stretcher on the ground, climb up and proceed forward with the stretcher. Now, the back portion of the stretcher is kept on the ground, the helpers climb up and again proceed.

4. While crossing the wall, both the front helpers keep the stretcher on the wall and climb up and get down on the other side and proceed forward. Now, the back helpers keep the stretcher on the wall and get down on the other side and proceed.

5. The stretcher is kept inside the ambulance with the head end ahead. Now, the two helpers go inside the ambulance and gently pull the stretcher inside, while the other two helpers, stand towards the foot end. When the whole stretcher gets inside the ambulance, it is fixed in position. While taking the stretcher out of the ambulance, two back helpers push the stretcher and the front two helpers pull and carry the whole stretcher to the full height of their arms to carry the patient to the bed in the hospital.

Lifting and carrying an injured person

If the helper is only one and the wound is minor

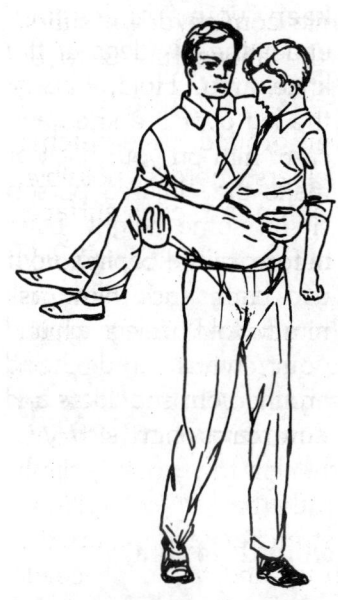

1. Method of carrying in hand/cradle

The method is used when the person is of less weight or is a child. In this method, the injured person should be carried from below the shoulder and knee with the hands. He should be carried comfortably.

Figure 72: The Cradle carry

2. Human crutch

In this method, the first aider himself stands near the injured person, holds his waist and keeps his hand on his neck, lift him with his another hand and takes him by giving him support.

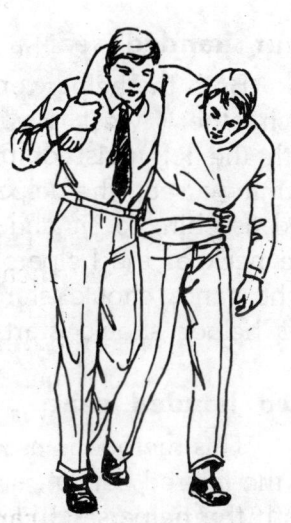

Figure 73.
The Human crutch

3. Fireman's lift

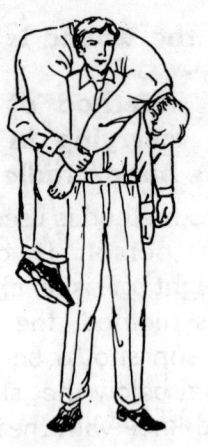

In this method, keep the injured person standing. Hold, one of his hand and keep your other hand under the two legs at the knee area. Hold, one of the leg over the knee and carry him on your back or make the injured person sit on some height, bend before him keeping your back at his face. Now, ask him to fold his legs around your waist. and hand around your shoulders and now carry him slowly.

Figure 74. The Fireman's Lift

If Helpers are two and wound is major

Four handed seat

Both the helper form a chair type seat by catching each other's wrist. Both helpers catch the right wrist with the left wrist of the other and vice-versa. After forming a seat, the helpers sit behind the injured person and ask him to sit and put both of his hands around the neck of the helpers. Now, the helper towards the right hand, should start with the right foot and the left helper should start with the left foot.

Two handed seat

This method is used when there is a hand fracture of the injured person, and he cannot catch the helpers. Both the helpers stand face to face by the side of the injured person and hold him by one hand from the chest line. Now, they lift him slightly and catch each

158

other's fingers by inserting hand from the middle portion of his thighs. The left side helper should keep his palm towards the upper side and the right side helper should keep his palm towards the down side by forming shape of hook with the help of fingers. Both should catch a hand kerchief or some cloth tightly. Now, both the helpers should start walking slowly.

The fore and AFT method

This method is used when there is no sufficient space for the use of chair. In this method, one helper catches the injured person only, putting his hands under the knees and the other helper catches him from encircling his chest. Both the helper carry the injured person, slowly.

On chair

In this method, the injured person is made to sit on a chair and is slowly carried by the helpers.

Blanket lift

If the injured person is lying on some bedsheet or blanket, then fold the bedsheet or blanket from both the sides or fold it by means of wooden rods. Now, the helpers should catch from all sides on the instruction of one of the helpers and should start walking slowly or if the stretcher is ready, then put the person on the stretcher and then carry him, give thick support of some cloth at the neck.

Improvised method

In this method, the button of the shirt of the injured person are opened and the open flaps of the shirt are folded and are caught by the helpers. The legs and head is held by other helpers and the person is made to lie on stretcher. The patient is covered by blanket and sand bag is kept by his neck sides.

If the hospital is far off or the ground is uneven, then the hips and knees should be tied with stretchers.

Loading and ambulance

A few ambulance have flat built in beds with grooves to take the runners of a standard stretcher. Four people are required to load this ambulance. One to stand inside the ambulance, ready to guide the stretcher. The other three stand on, one on either side of the stretcher and one at the end, ready to lift. If there are two berths, load the left one first.

Unloading the ambulance

One bearer catches the handles at the rear, while another person holds the handles at the head in the ambulance. The person at the back, gently withdraws the stretcher or trolley bed. After it is withdrawn, two bearers, one on each side of the trolley bed, support it, moving with side paces until the end is clear of the ambulance. The person in the ambulance, gets down, takes the handles at the head and helps to lower the trolley bed or stretcher to the ground.

Reef Knots

Always secure the ends of a bandage with a reef knot because it will not slip. It lies flat and is, therefore, move comfortable for the patient and it is easy to untie

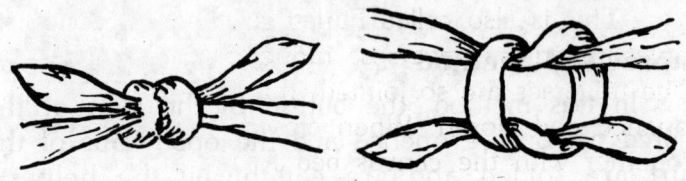

Figure 75. The Reef knot

160

Once the knot is tied, the ends should be tucked out of sight or neatly fastened to the bandage. Make sure that the knot does not press on to a bone or into the skin when used on a sling. If the knot is uncomfortable, place some soft padding under it.

First Aid Kits

While bandages and dressings can be improvised, it is better to have proper equipment on hand. These materials should be kept in clean, dry and airtight container. This should not be kept in a damp atmosphere, like, a bath room and be sure that it is clearly labeled.

A first aid kit should contain,

1. 10 individually wrapped sterile adhesive dressings
2. 1 sterile eye pad
3. 1 triangular bandage
4. 1 sterile covering for a serious wound.
5. 6 safety pins
6. 3 medium sized sterile dressings
7. 1 large sterile dressing
8. 1 extra large sterile dressing.

Different types of stretchers

1. The standard stretcher

This is also called Furley stretcher. It consists of poles, handles, traverses, runners and a canvas bed. The traverses are so jointed, that the stretcher can be opened and closed. When closed, the poles lie close together with the canvas bed folded at the top. This is, then, kept in position by two transverse straps. If strings are carried, they are laid along the canvas, held by the straps.

The stretcher can be opened thus, place the stretcher on its side with its runners towards you and the studs or buckles securing the straps upper most, unfasten any straps. Push the traverses fully open with your foot while placing the stretcher upright on the other end.

2. Closing the stretcher

Turn the stretcher on its side with its runners towards you. The studs or buckles which secure the straps uppermost. Push the joints of the traverses inwards with your heel to release them. Push the poles together, pulling the canvas out from between them. Canvas can be folded neatly on to the poles and secured with straps.

Scoop stretcher

The scoop or orthopaedic stretcher is an adjustable stretcher used to lift patients on to an ambulance trolley bed without altering the position in which they were found. It is not used to carry the patient too long distance. The length can be adjusted to suit any size of the patient and because he or she need not be moved. It is particularly useful for picking up the patient with a suspected spinal injury or internal injuries.

First, bring the stretcher to the patient's side and adjust the length. Then uncouple both ends of the stretcher and gently slip each half of the stretcher under the patient. The head sections should be rejoined. Place the head pad in position. When one first aider stays at the head, the other should rejoin the foot section. Secure the head pad to the stretcher. By working from either side of the stretcher, lift it and the patient and place on the trolley bed. The stretcher may be uncoupled and removed.

The fully adjustable stretcher bed on wheels is made of light metal and carried in many ambulances.

162

These trolley beds should always be kept ready for immediate use. A canvas sheet from a pole and canvas stretcher is placed on the stretcher bed and two blankets are placed on the top.

Utila folding stretcher

This is a light weight type of standard stretcher. It has light metal poles with telescopic handles and a canvas, or plastic bed. The folding stretcher is available in two ways. One folds in the same way as the standard stretcher. The other folds in half in the centre, and so, takes up less place.

Pole and canvas stretcher

This is the most commonly used stretcher. It has a canvas or plastic sheet about 200 cms long and 50 cms wide with two long poles. The canvas can be folded and slide under the patient. The poles are passed through sleeves, down the side of the canvas to form the stretcher. Spacer bars may be placed over the ends of the poles to keep them apart and the stretcher, firm.

Neil Robertson Stretcher

It is made of stout canvas and bamboo. This is designed for lifting patients in the upright position through small hatches like manholes or lowering the patients from heights, like in mountain rescue.

The patient is placed on the stretcher. The strap at top is passed around the patient's forehead to hold his head in position. The upperflaps are wrapped around the chest and secured with two short straps leaving the arms outside. The lower flaps are strapped round the lower limbs. The ring at the head of the stretcher is used for hoisting. The side rope rings should be used only for carrying by hand and should never be used as an aid to hoist the patient by ropes or lines. Another length of the rope is attached to the ring at the foot of the stretcher to guide it. The stretcher should be stored in a place where it is, most likely, to be needed together with a suitable length of rope, preferably, made of rot proof fibre.

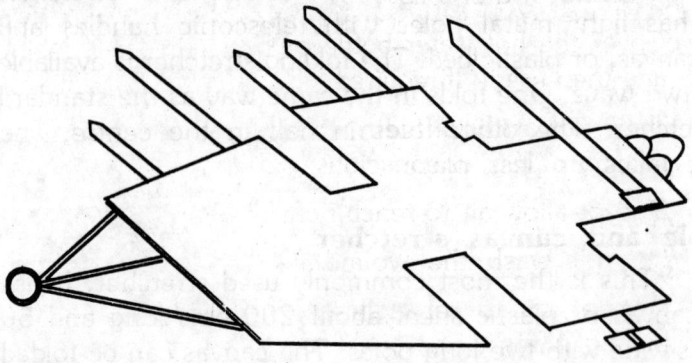

Figure 76. Neil Robertson Stretcher

Improvised stretchers

The broad-fold bandages at intervals around two strong poles. Spread out a ring, piece of sacking tarpaulin or a strong blanket and roll up two strong poles in the sides. Use a broad piece of wood, door or shutter and add a rug or straw covered with a piece of stout cloth or sacking. Turn the sleeves of two or three coats inside out. Pass two strong poles through sleeves and button up the coats.

Points to remember

1.   Do not touch any type of wound with finger or instruments.

2.   Do not keep dirty cloth or dressing on the wound.

3.   Do not allow the wound to bleed.

4.   Do not move the patient unnecessarily.

5.   Do not move the patient with the help of slings in a fracture.

6.   Do not ignore the condition of shock.

7.   Be careful, to see that the patient is not burnt with hot water bag.

8.   Cover the hot water bottle or bag with some cloth and then use it. If required, give artificial respiration.

9.   Take out artificial teeth, tobacco or pan from the mouth of an unconscious patient.

10. Do not allow air to reach near the burning clothes.

11. Do not wash the wound.

12. Do not try to set right the dislocated joints by pulling them.

13. Do not dress the wound with tobacco. Keep tourniquet loose.

14. Send some one to call the doctor.

Avoiding accidents on the road

Look straight in the direction you are going. Do not go anywhere, leaving the car in started condition. Do not peep out in the running car. Do not allow children to play near inflammable substances. Keep them beyond the reach of children. If the engine of the car is on and it is in the garage, do not keep the door closed. Pins, needles or any other sharp objects fallen on the floor, should be picked up immediately, as otherwise, children may get injured from them or even swallow them. Inflammable substances like petrol, gasoline etc. should be used with care.

FIRST AID AND EMERGENCY MANAGEMENT OF SPECIAL ORGANS

THE EYE

Affections of the eye due to injury or disease are very common and require careful and skillful treatment. Eye is a most delicate organ and even a slight injury is liable to be followed by unpleasant complications. So, all except a few minor cases should be treated by a doctor.

Red eyes

The condition is frequently diagnosed by the inexperienced as a cold or chill, but the inflammation is usually due to more serious cause such as, ulceration of the cornea or inflammation of the iris. This is beyond the scope of first aid.

Blows on the eye

Blows caused by tennis balls and similar objects may have serious consequences, even when the eye lids are closed, because the delicate structures within the eye ball, may be damaged and the back of the eye injured. The first aider should apply a pad and bandage and obtain medical advise as soon as possible.

166

The common result of the blow is what is called "Black eye". A cold compress secured tightly in position by a pad and bandage will often prevent a black eye, if applied early.

Perforating injuries

These are caused as a result of contact with pointed object as a spike. Partial rupture or even perforation of the eye ball is possible. A small wound appears and the pupil may become irregular. Part of the iris can be seen within the wound.

Foreign bodies in the eye

Foreign bodies, such as insects and pieces off grit or metal, often enter the eye and may be quite difficult to discover. They produce a feeling of discomfort and grittiness, which is accompanied by redness, congestion and watering. These symptoms and signs are similar to those caused by disease, and if, therefore, after a careful search, the first aider fails to discover a foreign body he must at once refer the patient to a doctor in case the trouble is due to a more serious condition such as an ulcer.

Examination and treatment

The patient should be comfortably seated, preferably in an easy-chair, with his head thrown backwards and suitably supported. The first aider should stand behind his patient and should examine the eye as follows:

1. Examination under lower lid

Instruct the patient to look upwards, and using the thumb, gently pull the lower lid downwards, drawing it away from the eyeball, so that its under surface can be examined. If the foreign body is not found in this situation, it is probably hidden under the upper eyelid, which must now be examined.

167

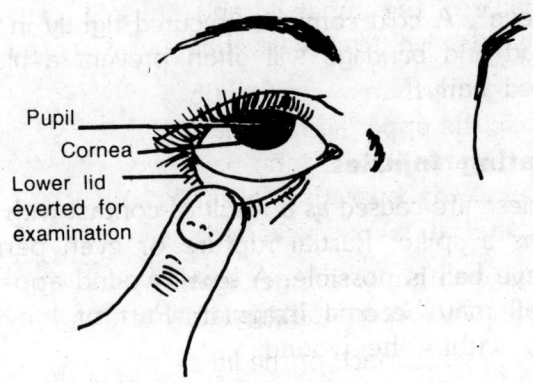

Pupil

Cornea

Lower lid
everted for
examination

Figure 77. Examination of lower lid

2. Examination under upper lid

This can only be undertaken when the eyelid is everted, i.e., turned inside out in such a way that its under surface is exposed. This process is painless and is undertaken as follows:

a) Reassure the patient that he will not feel pain and instruct him to look downwards. It is essential that he should keep looking downwards throughout the examination.

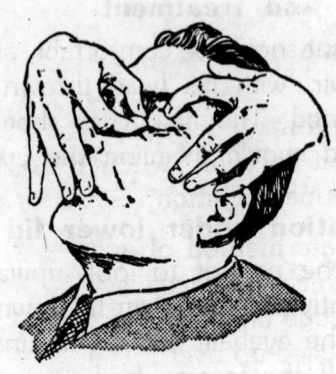

Figure 78. Everting the upper lid

168

b) Place the forefinger of the left hand upon the middle of the upper lid and press downwards and inwards, on to the eyeball.

c) Using the thumb and forefinger of the right hand, grasp the upper lid by its lashes and draw it slightly downwards towards the patient's cheek; then turn it upwards over the forefinger of the left hand so that it is now everted.

d) Remove the forefinger gently and instruct the patient to keep looking downwards.

The under surface of the lid can now be thoroughly examined.

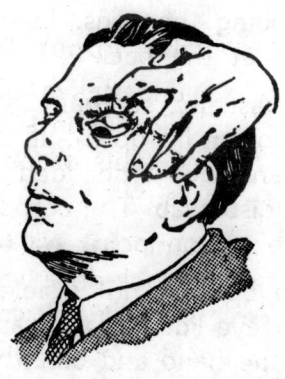

Figure 79. Upper lid everted for the examination

e) When the foreign body has been removed, instruct the patient to blink, when the eyelid will return to its normal position.

An alternate method of evertion involves the use of a match, which is placed across the lid about 12 mm above its edge and then pressed backwards as the eyelashes are pulled up over it. This method is precisely similar to that already suggested, except that the match replaced the forefinger.

169

3. Remove foreign body

When a foreign body is discovered under either of the lids, remove it by touching it with a wisp of cotton-wool or the twirled-up corner of a clean pocket-handkerchief which has been previously dampened with clean water.

4. Instill soothing drops

After removal of the foreign body, a few drops of castor oil should be placed within the eye and the patient warned that unless his symptoms quickly improve he should seek medical advice.

Management

1. Avoid rubbing the eyes. In case of a child, tie his hands at the back.

2. Seat the casualty, so that, light falls on the eye. Pull the lower lid down. If the foreign body is floating and not embedded, remove it with a narrow moist swab. The corner of a handkerchief twisted to a fine point will also do.

3. If foreign body is not visible, it may be under the upper eye lid. Ask the casualty to keep clean water in the hand and blink briskly in the water, if it is not gone pull, the upper lid forward, push the lower lid upwards and let go off both the lids. The lashes of lower lid, usually, dislodge the foreign body. Try this two or three times.

4. If the foreign body is embedded in the eye, particularly the cornea, do not touch it. Apply a soft pad, bandage the eye, ask the casualty not to rub the eye and take him immediately to a hospital.

5. Penetrating foreign bodies are easily made out by bleeding, pain etc., it is for the doctor to handle. You just put a pad and bandage.

THE EAR

There are four conditions liable to affect the ear. They are,

1. Haemorrhage or bleeding from the ear

It generally occurs when an ear drum ruptures or when the skull fracture is present. Bleeding from the ear channel may be caused by a laceration. Skull fractures are more serious and should be suspected if blood or clear watery cerebro spinal fluid mixed with blood is issuing from the ear.

If the bleeding is from the ear drum, there is pain in the ear, deafness and moderate flow of blood from the ear. If from within the skull, it may be due to skull fracture or head injury. The patient complains of head ache. Some blood mixed with clear watery cerebrospinal fluid may be coming from the ear. The patient may be unconscious.

The patient should be quickly removed to a hospital. If a skull fracture is suspected, pay attention to the level of responsiveness. All that is necessary is to apply a light dressing over the ear and bandage it in position. No attempt should be made to plug the canal. Small lacerations, if easily approachable, may be painted with an antiseptic. Otherwise, they should be left for medical attention. Transport as a stretcher, case maintaining the treatment position.

Foreign body in the ear

1. If it is an insect, fill the ear with glycerin or coconut/mustard oil or warm salt water. The insect will float up and can be removed easily.

2. If there is nothing floating up, leave it alone, do not meddle at all but take him to a doctor.

171

Ruptured ear-drum

This may be caused due to severe blows on the external ear. The condition may lead to bleeding in some cases.

First aid treatment include, applying a pad over the external ear and secure it with a bandage. Patient is made to lie down till he reach the hospital or seen by a doctor.

Ear-ache

The first aider should suspect of some foreign body in the ear. No treatment should be carried out unless seen by a doctor.

Ear blockage due to hardened wax

This may cause pain at times and also poor hearing.

The first aider should pull the pinna of the ear down and observe for hard wax. If confirmed, turn the patient head on the unaffected side, and pour few drops of coconut oil or olive oil, and allow it to absorb. The wax may become softened. Send the patient to the doctor for further treatment. Never pour water or irrigate the ear since this may cause damage of the ear-drum.

THE NOSE

Fractures, nose bleeding and foreign bodies are the three conditions commonly affecting the nose.

Fractures

The main problem associated with a nasal fracture is blockage of air way. So, every effort must be made to ensure that the patient has an open airway. A cold compress may give some relief. Treat any nose bleed and remove the patient to a hospital. Pain, swelling and bruising are usually present. The nose may appear

172

deformed and out of shape. Tenderness may be the only sign of a broken bone. In some cases, the chief injury is external. A broken nose is more serious than is commonly supposed and often requires a specialist for treatment. The first aider can only apply cold compresses and advise medical aid.

Nose bleeding

This is due to bleeding from the blood vessel inside the nostrils. It may occur due to a flow to the nose or the result of sneezing or blowing the nose. Watery looking blood stained fluid issuing from the nose may be a sign of a fractured skull. Nose bleeds can cause considerable loss of blood and may also cause the patient to swallow or inhale a great deal of blood. There may be vomiting and it may affect breathing.

There will be moderate flow of blood from nose. If there is skull fracture, there may be a mixture of blood and clear watery cerebro spinal fluid. High blood pressure during old age is also a cause of nose bleed. Small varicose veins are sometimes found inside the nose. These may rupture causing nose bleed. In some persons nose bleed occurs when he ascends to a high attitude. Nose bleeding, with discharge, in young children should always raise the suspicion that a foreign body may have pushed up the nose.

Make the patient sit down with her head well forward and loosen any tight clothing around her neck and chest. Advise the patient to breath through her mouth and to pinch the soft part of her nose. Do not allow the patient to talk, coughing, spitting or sniffing. Allow her to dribble and mop it up. Release the pressure after 10 minutes. If bleeding has not stopped, continue the process for another 10 minutes. Do not allow the patient to raise her head. While the head is still forward, get the patient clean around the nose gently with a swab or clean dressing soaked in luke warm water. Do not plug the nose. When the bleeding stops, tell the patient to avoid exertion and not to blow her nose for atleast 4 hours. If even after 30 minutes the bleeding has not stopped, seek medical aid.

Foreign body in the nose

Children often insert foreign bodies such as buttons and beads into the nose, usually the accident in quickly notified because the child itself calls attention.

First-aid measure

Unless it is obviously easy to remove the foreign, the first-aid should not try to remove. The child should be prevented from touching his nose and should be told to breathe through his mouth. If the child can co-operate, the child is asked to blow hard through his nose, keeping the sound nostril closed. The child should be warned not to inhale through his nose before blowing, to avoid the danger of drawing the foreign body further upwards.

THE THROAT

Foreign body in the throat

1. Some small objects, like a safety pin sometimes get struck in the throat. A drop of water is all, that is needed to pass in further down.

2. Some irregular objects, fairly large, get struck, if visible, they can be taken out with the fingers. If a child, hold it up, head downwards and tap on back and neck, the foreign body will fall out.

3. Fish bone or thorn get lodged by piercing some part of the throat. Keep the relatives and the casualty quiet and remove the casualty to the hospital at once.

174

Foreign body in the stomach

Smooth objects like coins, buttons, nuts, safety pins are swallowed.

1. The stomach and intestines will adjust themselves in such a way, as to throw them out.

2. Do not show any panic.

3. Show the case to the doctor.

4. There is no need to give laxatives.

Haemoptysis

Bleeding from the lungs is called haemoptysis. Usually, it indicates tuberculosis. It may occur due to complicated fractures of the ribs and by injury to the lungs. This may be a terminal event in acute pneumonia and secondary drowning.

The blood is generally bright red in colour and it is frothy, as it is mixed up with air. The blood is coughed up and the patient feels that it is coming from lungs. A sufferer from established tuberculosis will often be able to indicate the area of his lung which is affected by the disease.

The coughing up of blood causes great alarm to a patient. It is not usually dangerous and so the patient should reassured that it is not serious and the bleeding will stop. The patient must be advised to lie quite still in a darkened room which would provide both physical and mental relation. The patient should be made to lying down with his shoulders slightly raised. He should be turned towards the affected side, supported by pillows with head hanging down. This would prevent flooding of the affected parts of the lungs with blood. This position aids coughing. If there is shock, it should be treated by making the patient comfortable. Medical aid should immediately be obtained.

Haemetemesis

This is vomiting of blood. It is a disease of the stomach, like gastric ulcer or varicose veins. A patient who is about to have Haematemisis, will often exhibit symptoms and signs of shock and haemorrhage before the bleeding is actually visible. Blood from the stomach is vomited and is often mixed with undigested food. It is dark red in colour and may be clotted. If, however, blood has remained in the stomach for any length of time before vomiting actually occurs, it may partially be digested, in which case, it will have a coarse dark appearance. When the haemorrhage is due to gastric ulcer, a history of former dyspepsia is usually obtainable from the patient or his relatives.

Patient often does not realise that he is vomiting blood and for this reason when he is being reassured, there should be no reference to blood. Complete rest is essential in order to reduce bleeding to the minimum. It is important that the patient should remain lying down when vomiting is occurring. Nothing should be given by mouth except ice to suck. As far as possible, the patient should be kept lying down, with the feet raised and the head and shoulders low. Pillows should be removed. The services of a doctor should be obtained at the earliest possible moment.

Haemorrhage from the rectum

It may be due to local injury to the rectum itself as may occur in a complicated fracture of the pelvis. It may arise from diseases, like piles and ulceration of the bowel. A common cause of the bleeding is bleeding from duodenal ulcer. This variety is called "melaena".

The blood is of an ordinary red colour and is often mixed with a motion. Bleeding due to piles and ulcers in the bowel is rarely severe. It requires medical aid and not first aid measures. One of the commonest complications of a duodenal ulcer is bleeding inside the intestines. Then blood passes throughout the digestive tract, and finally, causing melaen. The usual symptoms, signs of shock and haemorrhage are present. The blood which is passed from the rectum is of dark red in colour or even black, like tar.

Uterine haemorrhage

Haemorrhage from the uterus, apart from natural bleeding, may be due to disease to a threatened miscarriage.

Haematuria

Bleeding from any part of urinary tract shows itself in urine and is known haematuria. It may be from injury or disease of any of the organs comprising the genito urinary system.

Patients suffering from bleeding, however slight, from rectum, stomach, lungs, bladder etc. should see a doctor without delay, so that, the cause may be investigated.

Contusion

Slight bleeding under the skin resulting from violence, causes a bruise or contusion. This may be treated by the use of an evaporating lotion or by the application of a pressure bandage.

EMERGENCY CARE IN DISASTERS AND FIRST AID

Disasters

Disasters are sudden, catastrophic events that disrupt patterns of life, in which, there is possible loss of life and property in addition to multiple injuries. Disaster means, an adverse or unfortunate event or a great and sudden misfortune. The common elements of any disaster are casualties, homeless persons, disruption of sanitary facilities, some degree of panic, and need for emergency medical services. The people affected by any such event are panic struck and they need first aid care, emergency treatment, food, shelter, clothing and the basic requirements of life, which are not easily available in such circumstances.

Types of disasters

1. **Natural disasters:** Flood or drought, wind storm (cyclone or hurricane) earth quake or volcanic eruption, epidemic.

2. **Man made unintentional disasters:** Fire, explosion, accidents of trains, aircrafts or ships.

3. **Intentional disasters:** Ordinary bombing, atomic bombing, biologic warfare, chemical warfare.

Responsibilities of Health workers

During disaster, the sick persons need ingenuity and imagination to utilize things which are available at hand, these have so much responsibility during such times of stress.

1. She should provide them medical and nursing care and she should look after the injured and sick persons.

2. She should give constant observation and treatment to seriously wounded person to arrest the bleeding and to save the life.

3. She should take measure to check the infection.

4. She should maintain the sanitation and cleanliness around the place of relief.

5. Arrange to put up a temporary shelter place quickly.

6. She should arrange the initial examination and health check up of all those coming to the relief centre.

7. Arrange the nutritional facilities to the injured, children and infants.

8. Arrange them for drinking water, give special care to the pregnant mothers, infants, old age people, people with other problems.

9. She should arrange for transporting them immediately to the hospital or health centres.

10. Make arrangement to intimate to their relatives, as early as possible.

Aspects of relief work in disasters

During disaster, the number of people will be its victim and whether they die or are crippled, will depend to a great extent on how well the community and its homes are prepared to meet such emergencies. Nowadays, thermo nuclear warfare is considered to be ultimate type of disaster but the local community striken by storm, fire, earthquake, or explosion may well face almost as high casualty rates as would be the nation in case of nuclear war. A village inundated by flood with a loss of over 4,000 lives is devastated as severely as if, it were hit by a bomb.

What happens to the average community or family in a disaster area? First of all, the electric power supply is impaired. Without electricity, there are no lights, radio and television station will no longer function. The telephone lines may well be out of operation making it difficult to summon help from the fire or police departments or to contact the family physician or local hospital. Even if they can be contacted, the condition of the roads and streets may make it impossible for them to reach you. If the grocery store faces the disaster, their contents may be so damaged to be unsafe to use. The water of many communities is pumped from a well, reservoir or lake by electric pumps. If the pumping station is damaged, the water supply will quickly be exhausted or the disaster may damage water mains so badly that contamination makes the water no longer safe.

Disease thrives under disaster condition. Prevention of disease, involves sanitation, isolation and immunization.

Sanitation involves the proper disposal of waste, especially, human waste and the control of whatever may carry disease. Disease carries include, rodents, house flies, mosquitoes and other insects.

Isolation refers to the process by which the individual with a communicable disease is kept separated from healthy individual, as nearly as possible, to prevent the spread of his disease. Isolation is always not easy under disaster conditions but may always be carried out to a certain degree. The person who covers his mouth while coughing is practicing isolation.

Immunization is the best form of preventive medicine, it is, especially, practical step in preparing for disaster situation because it can be taken in advance.

Every community should have a civil defence plan and orgnisation. This can be used not only for nuclear attack, but also, for any other kind of disaster. For effective and successful relief work in disasters, doctors, nurses para medical people, police, military and other volunteers must participate.

_____

UNIT 13

COMMUNITY EMERGENCIES

Disaster management

Remember : An important principle is "Do not further harm".

Be conscious of your own safety. Do not place your own life in jeopardy. The most immediate concern are lack of breathing and haemorrhage which if not controlled will lead to death.

The first-aider may be the first on the scene to assess the disaster and initiate the mass disaster plan. This means alerting your department to the type of disaster and number of casualties, which allows preplanned notifications to be made. Notification includes the hospital, other public safety agencies.

Community emergencies

1. Fire explosions

This is one of the disasters seen in the community. The fire explosions either due to electrical leakage or blasts can cause considerable damage to the buildings and surroundings where the people are dwelling.

During the disaster, the first aider should attend to the following needs -

a) Put off the main electrical line of fire is caused due to electricity.

b) Evacuate the victims from the house/building as early as possible.

c) If the victirns are suffocated treat them accordingly.

d) Attend to the minor burns.

e) In case of major burns, treat for shock, if any, first, and send or accompany the victims to the nearby hospital for further treatment.

f) Inform legal authorities regarding the type and occurrence of fire-explosions.

g) In case of the explosion is of greater nature call for help from Fire-fighting service who can help you in evacuating the victim from the place of fire-explosion.

II. Floods

This disaster is commonly seen during summer or rainy season and the people living near either side seashore or low lying areas. Flood always has a warning signal. In case of floods, the dwellers should be evacuated to a safer place and the first aider , as fast as possible should try to minimize the damage going to happen to life and property.

Young children required special attention and should be rescued first from drowning due to flood waters. Adults, and aged must be helped to get into a safe place.

In case the person drowned are treated with the first-aid measures taken routinely for drowning and asphyxia.

183

If the victim require hospital management they should be sent to nearby health centres/hospitals for further treatment. Meanwhile help is taken from the concerned authorities, police and sometimes even divers to save the people who have drowned.

III. Earthquakes

Earthquakes is a disaster which occur without prior significance. In a major earthquake the victims number may go substantially high and which may include the conditions such as head injuries, fractures, unconsciousness, minor injuries and even deaths. A first-aider who witnesses the earthquake should be alert specially is isolating the victims and attending to the serious victims first according to priority. A helping squad from the nearby hospital should be summoned in case of medical team arrive late. The victim who need hospital management should be sent/ or accompanied to the hospital.

The victims are given first-aid treatment according to the type of episode occurred. Eg: Head injuries, unconsciousness etc. The first-aider should record all the observations on the patient and brief report may accompany to the patient to the hospital.

IV. Famine

Famine is a disaster caused by the nature. The first-aider in cases of famine should contact the voluntary or government agencies to get assistance which may be in the field of either food or shelter or both. The first-aider can also help in arranging immediate requirement such as drinking water, milk, bread or other staple food from the nearby places or through some voluntary agencies.

Rehabilitation

Rehabilitation of vulnerable weak classes in the above disasters require top priority beyond the condition

184

become worse. The first-aider should have ready in hand informations regarding to different rehabilitation centres for different categories for disasters.

The rehabilitation should include

a) Providing food for the victims
b) Basic medical care
c) Schooling for children
d) Provision of clothing
e) Housing
f) Financial assistance
g) Providing jobs to earn their livelihood.
h) Supervision from the social service department including psychological support.

Community resources

Police assistance

In almost all the disasters, the police assistance may be of much importance to protect the life and property of people in addition to maintaining the law and order situation. The first-aider should contact the local police force for any kind of help and suggestion, either in controlling the mob, direct to individual to proper area, or in providing the basic needs of the victims.

The first-aider and the police force should work as a team in cases of disaster to avert any untoward incident occurring following the disasters. The police force itself is trained and equipped with personnel to meet any challenge at this time of crisis. Therefore, the police assistance is of great help to a first-aider.

Ambulance service

Transport is the prompt and safe moving of the patient from the emergency scene to a medical facility, providing emergency care and gathering information while enroute.

185

Ambulances are nowadays fitted with radio communications to hospitals. The ambulance should have all facilities to meet any eventuality during the transport of the patient.

This includes:

a) Stretchers

b) Oxygen administration apparatus

c) B.P. apparatus

d) I.V. infusion stand

d) Emergency drugs

f) Airway

g) Pillows

h) Towels

i) Stethoscope

The first-aider should accompany the victim to the hospital preferably with a trained nurse who can handle the equipment and monitor the patient effectively.

The ambulance should have the necessary "Logo" and Bell system to have easy access to the hospital on the way. The nearest route may be used to reach the hospital. The victim and one of his relative may be permitted in the ambulance.

The first-aider if accompany the victim should check the patient vital sign and other condition very often till the victim is reached to the hospital or to a medical practitioner.

In case of death while transporting the victim to the hospital, the first-aider should take the ambulance to the hospital to get the "certificate of death" from the Doctor. The first-aider should give a detailed report of the victim regarding condition at the time of disaster and till he reaches to the hospital.

International agencies

WHO

World Health Organization (WHO) which is a specialized non-political health agency of the United Nations with headquarters in Geneva was established in 1946.

The objective of the WHO is "The Attainment by all people of the highest level of health."

WHO assists in many projects related to health and assists in developing education both medical and nursing. It also assists Epidemiological survey on Communicable diseases. The WHO has also paid attention, in the programme of work to Non-communicable disease problems such as cancer, cardiovascular diseases, genetic disorders, mental disorders, drug addiction and dental diseases. Promotion of environmental health has always been important an activity of the World Health Organization.

WHO advises Government or National programmes keeping pace with the health requirement.

UNICEF

UNICEF (United Nations Children's Emergency Fund) is one of the specialized agencies of the United Nations. It was established in 1946. UNICEF works in close relationship with WHO and looksafter the welfare of Children both in preventive and curative aspects of disease.

FAO

The Food and Agricultural Organization (FAO) was found in 1945 with headquarters in Rome.

The main aims of FAO are -

1. To help nations to raise living standards.

2. To improve nutrition of the people.

3. To increase the efficiency in farming, forestry and fisheries.

4. To better the conditions of rural people.

Non-governmental and other agencies

1. **Rockfellar foundation :** Is a philosophical organization. The main work at present include agriculture, family planning and rural training centres.

2. **Ford foundation :** Is responsible to develop orientation training centres, research cum action projects and pilot projects in rural health scheme.

3. **CARE (Co-operative in American Relief Everywhere) :** It is responsible to provide mobile health care and advice.

International Red Cross

The Red Cross is a non-political, non-official international humanitarian organization devoted to the service of mankind both during peace and war. It was founded by Henry Dunant.

Red Cross provide service in disasters, wars and major casualties. It also helps to provide education in First-aid and nursing, health education and maternity and child welfare services.